CW00631870

Pathophysiology of
the Nervous System

$\frac{12}{+p}$ £18.95

Pathophysiology of the Nervous System

Lewis Sudarsky, M.D.

Assistant Professor of Neurology, Harvard Medical School; Assistant Chief, Neurology Service, VA Medical Center, West Roxbury; Associate in Neurology, Beth Israel Hospital, and Brigham and Women's Hospital, Boston

With a contribution by

Stephen L. Hauser, M.D.

Associate Professor of Neurology, Harvard Medical School; Director, Immunology Unit, Massachusetts General Hospital, Boston

Foreword by

Martin A. Samuels, M.D.

Associate Professor of Neurology, Harvard Medical School; Chief, Neurology Division, Brigham and Women's Hospital, Boston

Little, Brown and Company
Boston/Toronto/London

Copyright © 1990 by Lewis Sudarsky

First Edition

All rights reserved. No part of this book may be reproduced in any form or by any electronic or mechanical means, including information storage and retrieval systems, without permission in writing from the publisher, except by a reviewer who may quote brief passages in a review.

Library of Congress Catalog Card No. 90-61712

ISBN 0-316-82117-9

Printed in the United States of America

RRD-VA

Cover illustration reprinted by permission of the publishers from *The Post Natal Development of the Cerebral Cortex*, Vol. VI, by Jesse LeRoy Conel, Harvard University Press, Copyright © 1959 by the President and Fellows of Harvard College.

Contents

Foreword

I have spent a large proportion of my career teaching neurology—teaching it to medical students, neurology residents, residents in other fields, and postgraduate physicians, neurologists, and non-neurologists. One notices a paradox in trying to teach this discipline. On the one hand, the subject is inherently interesting, attracting the initial attention of the student. On the other hand, as the complexity of the basic science underlying the clinical practice increases, the interest of the student rapidly wanes. Many students, regardless of their stage of life, feel they simply cannot understand clinical neurology, partly because of intellectual intimidation and partly because the ante is simply too high: too much neuroanatomy, neurophysiology, neuropharmacology, neurogenetics, and neuropathology prior to the rewards of diagnosing and treating a patient. With the dramatic professionalization of the neurosciences, this paradox has become all the more vivid. Perhaps the next great frontier in medical science involves unlocking the mysteries of the nervous system, but can a regular medical doctor share in the fun?

The secret to teaching this discipline is to take advantage of the first phase of fascination, during which one can transmit the superstructure upon which all of neurologic knowledge is based. This involves understanding the major principles of neuroanatomy, neurophysiology, and neuropharmacology upon which the details can later be added. In *Pathophysiology of the Nervous System*, Dr. Lewis Sudarsky demonstrates his experience as a celebrated teacher of neurology at Harvard. This book is something we have been seeking for many years: a textbook for the introductory course in pathophysiology of the nervous system. In addition, the book can serve as a reintroduction to neurology for generations of medical students past who were alienated by the fact density of prior approaches to this subject. My only fear is that this eloquently written, crystal-clear exposition will result in a glut of applications to our neurologic residencies, most of which I have to review.

Martin A. Samuels, M.D.

Preface

There has been an explosion of knowledge in the neurosciences in the past decade. The excitement resonates through the applied fields of neurology and psychiatry. At the same time, the velocity of change has stressed the capacity of the best physician to keep up. To some degree, neuroscience and the related clinical disciplines have become separate cultures. *Pathophysiology of the Nervous System* was written for second- and third-year medical students. It attempts to bridge the widening gap between the basic sciences and the culture of clinical medicine. It may also be of use to older students, residents, even practicing physicians as a review and update. We tried to produce a book that was compact and manageable, with clinical emphasis and a contemporary neuroscience perspective.

The half-life of medical information is short, and much of what we presently know about diseases of the nervous system will soon be out of date. In recognition of this fact, we have given *pathophysiology* a liberal interpretation. Rather than writing a detailed treatment on the mechanisms of disease, we have focused on presenting a conceptual framework. We have tried to give a view of the nervous system, a picture of its workings and its vulnerabilities. Disease mechanisms are considered in more detail where they complement the picture. In the presentation, we have tried to acknowledge the source and development of existing ideas.

The study of nervous system disorders has an added dimension in neuroanatomy. The anatomic bias of the neurologic examination attests to the importance of anatomy in clinical thinking. We are trained to ask first, Where is the lesion? The ability to do an examination and make a localization at the bedside are powerful tools, which the student must master. This is not primarily a book about anatomy or about clinical skills. But it was impossible to ignore neuroanatomy in writing a book of this nature. I hope that the consideration here of certain anatomic topics contributes rather than detracts.

Several topics were not included. The neurology of the special senses (the visual system, hearing, and balance) is an important subject that was just too big to put into a small book. There is no separate chapter on neurogenetics. It is a highly specialized topic, one that is often given separate consideration with genetics in a medical school curriculum. Yet we decided to include a chapter on immunology and virology of the nervous system because an understanding of this material is essential for contemporary clinical practice.

The book is organized into four parts. The first part, Nerve, Muscle, and Synapse, explores the motor unit. It provides a foundation for understanding neuromuscular disease. The second part, Sensory-Motor Integration, considers pain and somatic sensation, as well as the organization of movement. These chapters provide a systems level approach to neurology. Part III is about cortical functions: disorders of consciousness, epilepsy, and behavioral neurology. Finally, Vulnerabilities of the Nervous System considers the brain and spinal cord as an organ system, together with some of the diseases to which they are prone. This part considers issues such as stroke, brain tumor, head trauma, viral infection, and demyelinating disease.

Several people participated in this project, and I would like to acknowledge their help. The list begins with Frisso Potts and Marty Samuels, colleagues who helped with the development of the book. Carole Warkel and Janet Miele helped with typing and preparation. The editorial staff at Little, Brown was a consistent source of encouragement and assistance. I also want to thank Marty Samuels and Charles Barlow for their support while this was "in the works."

L. S.

Pathophysiology of

the Nervous System

PART I

Nerve, Muscle, and Synapse

NOTICE. The indications and dosages of all drugs in this book have been recommended in the medical literature and conform to the practices of the general medical community. The medications described do not necessarily have specific approval by the Food and Drug Administration for use in the diseases and dosages for which they are recommended. The package insert for each drug should be consulted for use and dosage as approved by the FDA. Because standards for usage change, it is advisable to keep abreast of revised recommendations, particularly those concerning new drugs.

CHAPTER 1

Nerve

The peripheral nervous system (PNS) is an extensive network, an information utility. It services the muscles and cutaneous sense organs distributed throughout the body wall. Peripheral nerves carry frequency-coded messages to and from centers of information processing in the brainstem and spinal cord. Figure 1-1 details the location of the major nerves in the limbs. The ulnar nerve is palpable as it winds through the ulnar groove under the elbow (the "funny bone"). The common peroneal nerve can be palpated behind the knee, along the fibular head.

What's inside a nerve? A mixed nerve is primarily a cable with myelinated and unmyelinated axons, efferents, and sensory afferents. Intermixed with the axons are Schwann cells, each of which provides myelin to a segment of a single axon. The excitable tissue is surrounded by a tough fibrous sheath, the epineurium, an extension of the dura mater. Perineurium and endoneurium beneath invest individual fascicles of nerve (Fig. 1-2). The basal lamina of the nerve sheath provides a guide for peripheral nerve regeneration after injury. The nerve has its own arterial plexus, the vasa nervorum. Specializations at the capillary level form a barrier to large molecules, similar to the blood-brain barrier of the central nervous system (CNS).

The axons within a mixed nerve vary with regard to fiber diameter. Some of the smallest fibers lack myelin (or contain it in minimal amounts). Figure 1-3 is a teased fiber histogram, which displays the contents of a mixed nerve. The unmyelinated fibers are 0.5 to 2.0 μm in diameter, while the largest fibers, the Ia afferents, average 8 to 12 μm. Detailed studies of axon populations indicate that diseases of the PNS have characteristic patterns of injury. In amyloid neuropathy, for example, depopulation of small, unmyelinated fibers is observed. These fibers are primarily pain afferents and autonomic efferents.

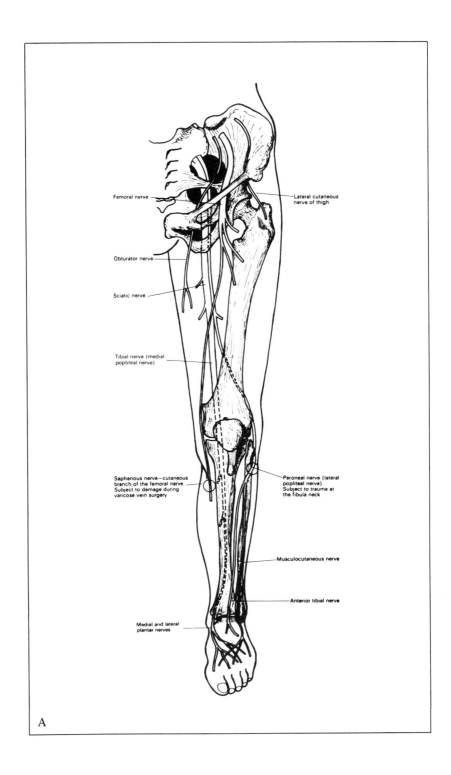

A

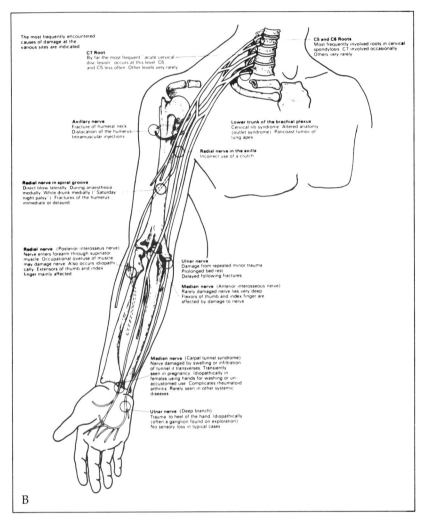

The most frequently encountered
causes of damage at the
various sites are indicated

C7 Root
By far the most frequent "acute cervical
disc lesion" occurs at this level. C6
and C5 less often. Other levels very rarely

C5 and C6 Roots
Most frequently involved roots in cervical
spondylosis. C7 involved occasionally.
Others very rarely

Axillary nerve
Fracture of humeral neck
Dislocation of the humerus
Intramuscular injections

Lower trunk of the brachial plexus
Cervical rib syndrome. Altered anatomy
(outlet syndrome). Pancoast tumor of
lung apex

Radial nerve in the axilla
Incorrect use of a crutch

Radial nerve in spiral groove
Direct blow laterally. During anaesthesia
medially. While drunk medially ("Saturday
night palsy"). Fractures of the humerus
immediate or delayed

Radial nerve (Posterior interosseus nerve)
Nerve enters forearm through supinator
muscle. Occupational overuse of muscle
may damage nerve. Also occurs idiopathically. Extensors of thumb and index
finger mainly affected

Ulnar nerve
Damage from repeated minor trauma
Prolonged bed rest
Delayed following fractures

Median nerve (Anterior interosseous nerve)
Rarely damaged nerve lies very deep
Flexors of thumb and index finger are
affected by damage to nerve

Median nerve (Carpal tunnel syndrome)
Nerve damaged by swelling or infiltration
of tunnel it transverses. Transiently
seen in pregnancy. Idiopathically in
females using hands for washing or un-
accustomed use. Complicates rheumatoid
arthritis. Rarely seen in other systemic
diseases

Ulnar nerve (Deep branch)
Trauma to heel of the hand. Idiopathically
(often a ganglion found on exploration)
No sensory loss in typical cases

B

FIGURE 1-1 (Continued).

FIGURE 1-1. The nerve supply to the extremities is summarized in these two figures. Points of vulnerability are noted, where nerves are adjacent to ligaments or bone. (From J. Patten, *Neurological Differential Diagnosis*. New York: Springer-Verlag, 1983, pp. 196, 209, with permission.)

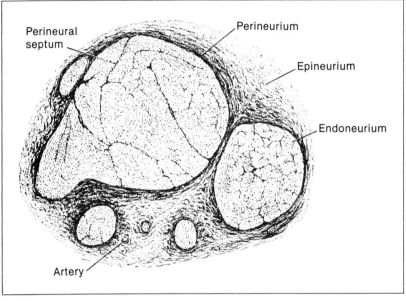

FIGURE 1-2. The fibrous layers which surround a peripheral nerve are seen in this cross section of the monkey sciatic nerve. The mixed nerve is invested by epineurium. Fascicles are surrounded by perineurium; endoneurium is the intrafascicular connective tissue. (From M.B. Carpenter and J. Sutin, *Human Neuroanatomy* [8th ed]. Baltimore: Williams & Wilkins, 1985, p. 185, with permission.)

NERVE IMPULSE TRANSMISSION

The principal function of nerve is the faithful transmission of electrical signals. Specializations of the axon cylinder which permit this function include its lipid membrane, which is relatively impermeable to aqueous solution, and ion channels. A detailed derivation of the membrane basis of the action potential is outside the scope of this chapter, but we will review the essential details in brief.

Resting potential is produced by the separation of charge across the membrane. Cations (sodium and potassium) leak out and accumulate near the cell surface membrane. A voltage potential difference, negative by about 70 mV on the inside, opposes the diffusion of additional potassium ions down their concentration gradient out of the cell. The membrane potential is thus at or near the equilibrium potential for potassium (the difference being due to the small traffic in sodium ions). Small ion currents of sodium (inward) would ultimately result in equilibration, dissipating the membrane potential. This "battery

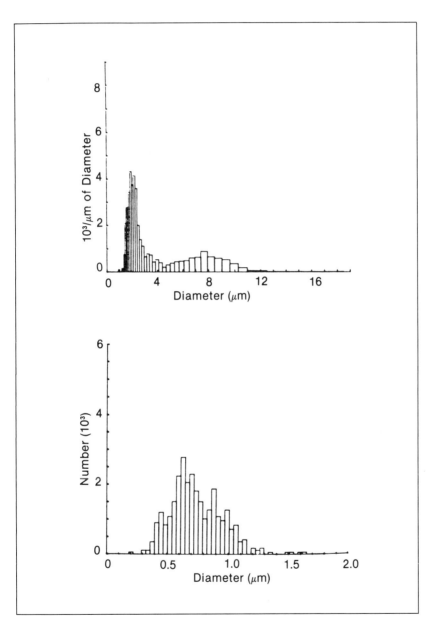

FIGURE 1-3. Histogram displays contents of myelinated (*top*) and unmyelinated (*bottom*) fibers from a fascicular biopsy specimen of human sural nerve. The histogram shows the distribution of fibers by size. Note the bimodal distribution of myelinated fibers. The largest myelinated fibers (8–12 μm) are fast-conducting, corresponding to the Ia afferents. (From E. Lambert and P. Dyck, *Peripheral Neuropathy*. Philadelphia: Saunders, 1975, p. 432, with permission.)

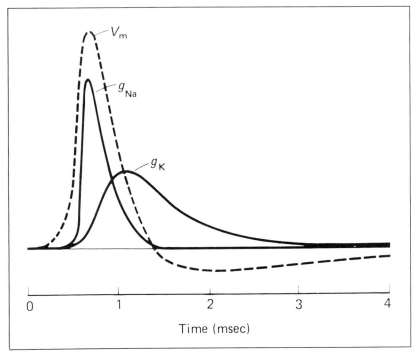

FIGURE 1-4. The ionic events which underlie the action potential are displayed here as a function of time. V_m denotes the course of the membrane potential. g_{Na} and g_K denote the membrane permeability to sodium and potassium, respectively. Opening of voltage-gated sodium channels initiates the rapid rise in the action potential. Closing of sodium channels and opening of the potassium channels cause the repolarization and late hyperpolarization (From E.R. Kandel and J.H. Schwartz [eds.], *Principles of Neural Science* [2nd ed.]. New York: Elsevier, 1985, with permission.)

run-down" does not occur because it is countered by the Na^+-K^+ pump. This energy-dependent mechanism preserves the membrane concentration gradients in an optimal state for signal transmission.

The action potential is generated by a transient alteration in membrane permeability. The explosive and self-propagating nature of the action potential is due to a built-in positive feedback mechanism: the voltage-gated sodium channel. Initially, a change in membrane potential (caused by postsynaptic potentials or a large signal potential upstream) opens sodium channels, resulting in an abrupt inward current of sodium ions. The current produces further depolarization, and more sodium channels open. As a large number of sodium ions pour into the cell, the membrane potential rises to approach the equilibrium potential for sodium (roughly +55 mV). The action potential has two late events which limit the depolarization: (1) After a time, sodium channels are inactivated, and (2) potassium channels open in the middle of the cycle. This liberates an outward potassium current, which tends to repolarize and even hyperpolarize the membrane (Fig. 1-4).

A toxin produced by the puffer fish (suborder Tetraodontoidea) specifically blocks the axon sodium channel. Tetrodotoxin is useful in the study of neuronal membrane physiology in the laboratory. The poisonous fish inhabits the seas of the Indian Ocean and South Pacific. Exposure to its toxin causes conduction block and paralysis, such that the puffer fish has few natural predators. The fish is nonetheless a delicacy enjoyed by a traditional cult in Japan. The toxin is largely inactivated by steaming, but the ritual has an occasional casualty.

The speed of transmission of the action potential along the axon is determined by its passive cable properties, particularly axon diameter. Depolarization causes an ion current to run along the inside of the cell. The spread of the ionic current is limited by the internal resistance of the axoplasm and the leakage of current through the membrane. The speed of propagation of the action potential is inversely proportional to the product of the internal resistance and the membrane capacitance. An increase in diameter will greatly reduce the internal resistance, and speed transmission. Consequently the large-diameter Ia afferents in peripheral nerve have the fastest conduction velocity.

Myelin

Myelin is another specialization which has evolved to facilitate rapid signal transmission. The lipid layers which wrap around the axon like a jelly roll decrease the capacitance of the membrane, and limit the leakage of current. The relation between conduction velocity and fiber diameter for myelinated and unmyelinated nerves is depicted in Figure 1-5.

Voltage-gated sodium channels are concentrated at the internode, each 1 to 2 mm in diameter. Regeneration of the action potential at the internodes is necessary to keep the signal going. This process is often referred to as *saltatory conduction,* though the action potential spans up to 100 nodes at any time. By limiting the diffusion of ions and the dissipation of the current, the myelin sheath increases the metabolic efficiency of the axon per unit length. This arrangement also facilitates miniaturization in the peripheral nervous system. The long distance from spinal cord to distal limb in vertebrate species demands fast transmission times. Without myelination, axons of enormous diameter

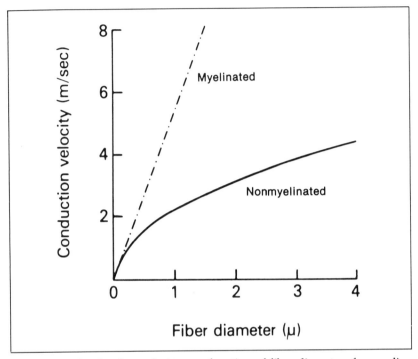

FIGURE 1-5. Conduction velocity as a function of fiber diameter, for myelinated and unmyelinated fibers. Conduction occurs more rapidly in a myelinated axon than in an unmyelinated axon of comparable size. (From S.G. Waxman and M.V. Bennett, Relative conduction velocities of small myelinated and non-myelinated fibers in the central nervous system. *Nature* 238 : 217, 1972, with permission.)

would be required. We will consider below the functional consequences that occur when axons lose their myelin sheath due to disease.

Axoplasmic Transport

In addition to electrical signals, material substance is passed along the axon. Neurons have a transport system, which moves cytoplasmic contents down the nerve from cell body to nerve terminal. A fast axoplasmic transport system carries proteins and other macromolecules along the internal cytoskeleton at about 400 mm/day. A slow axoplasmic transport, probably a bulk flow mechanism, proceeds at 1 to 3 mm/day carrying neurofilaments and organelles. A retrograde transport system has also been demonstrated, the speed of which is roughly 150 to 200 mm/day.

Nerve terminals appear to have a trophic function on the tissues they innervate. Dramatic changes are observed in skeletal muscle fibers after a loss of innervation. Acetylcholine receptors become more diffuse in the membrane, and other postsynaptic specializations are lost. Trophic factors are thought to influence many of these nerve–target cell interactions. Axoplasmic flow may be important in maintaining the presynaptic reserve of peptides and trophic factors.

REACTIONS OF NERVE

What happens when there is "loss of nerve?" A large number of diseases affect the peripheral nervous system, but a limited number of response patterns characterize the tissue. The diseases of peripheral nerve produce a few common syndromes. Consequently, when patients present with a diffuse disorder of peripheral nerve, it is often difficult to make a specific diagnosis. A good neurologist will make a proper etiologic diagnosis in about 60 percent of cases, while a specialist in peripheral nerve disorders may diagnose 75 to 80 percent after extensive testing. This still leaves a large number of cases unresolved. (Even nerve biopsy is commonly a nondiagnostic procedure.)

Wallerian Degeneration

Figure 1-6 illustrates wallerian degeneration, the response of a neuron when its axon is severed. Deprived of nourishment and other maintenance by axoplasmic transport, the axon degenerates distal to the point of interruption. There is also disintegration of peripheral myelin within the bounds of the endoneurium. Blocks or ovoids are observed to contain axon fragments. Retrograde changes are observed in the neuron soma. A dissolution of Nissl substance occurs in the nerve cell body (central chromatolysis) as the neuron prepares to regrow axon. With very proximal lesions, there is a reduction in the dendritic tree and a distinct chance that the cell may die. Otherwise, regeneration of the distal axon proceeds, provided the nerve sheath layers are not interrupted. After nerve injury, a severed axon will generally regrow its distal process at a rate of 1 mm/day over a period of months.

Peripheral Neuropathy

A long list of diseases affects nerve tissue diffusely, producing a syndrome known as *peripheral neuropathy* (Table 1-1). This is a common syndrome in clinical practice. Deficits are distal, and are appreciated first in the lower extremities, later in the fingertips. Patients often complain of paresthetic numbness ("pins and needles"); sometimes

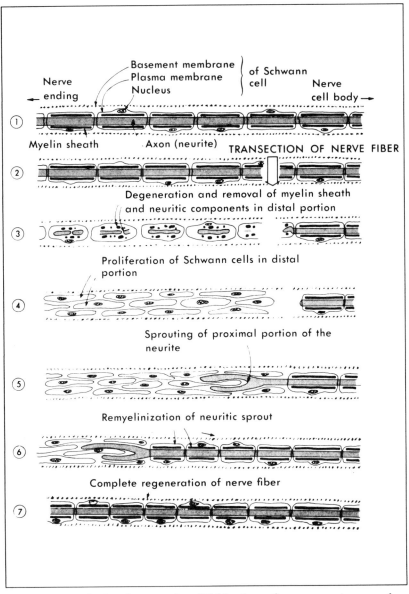

FIGURE 1-6. Wallerian degeneration: Within days after an axon is severed (2), there is distal degeneration of the axon and fragmentation of the myelin sheath. Proximal changes in the cell body are not illustrated. Schwann cells proliferate distally in preparation for regeneration (4). Sprouting occurs, with slow growth and remyelination of the regenerating nerve fiber (5–7). (From R. Escourolle and J. Poirier, *Manual of Basic Neuropathology*, L. Rubenstein [trans.]. Philadelphia: Saunders, 1971, p. 193, with permission.)

TABLE 1-1. Causes of Peripheral Neuropathy

Metabolic
Diabetes
Uremia
Porphyria
Hypothyroidism
Chronic liver disease

Nutritional
Thiamine deficiency
Vitamin B_{12} deficiency
Pyridoxine deficiency
Mixed B vitamin deficiency
Malabsorbtion

Drugs and toxins
Lead, arsenic, mercury, thallium
Isoniazid
Nitrofurantoin
Disulfiram
Phenytoin
Chloroquine
Vincristine
Acrylamide
Organophosphates
Trichloroethylene, carbon disulfide
Other hydrocarbon solvents

Infectious
Leprosy
Diphtheria

Immune
Guillain-Barré syndrome
Chronic inflammatory polyneuropathy
Vasculitis
Dysproteinemias

Paraneoplastic
Subacute sensory neuropathy

Genetically determined
Hereditary sensorimotor neuropathy (types I, II, III)
Amyloidosis
Refsum's disease

---

the condition is painful. There is a "stocking-and-glove" pattern of sensory loss. Weakness and loss of reflex may be observed in distal muscles. All these manifestations derive from length-dependent failure of nerve function. Two principal mechanisms (patterns of injury) are observed.

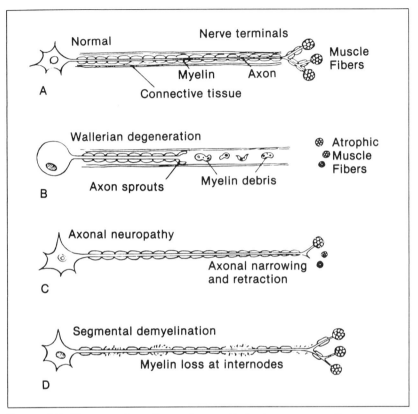

FIGURE 1-7. Figure reviews the various pathologic processes affecting peripheral nerve. In axonal neuropathy, as in wallerian degeneration, there is distal degeneration of the myelin and axis cylinder. Muscle atrophy occurs as a consequence of denervation. In segmental demyelination, the axon is spared, and no trophic changes are observed in skeletal muscle. (From J. Daube et al., *Medical Neurosciences* [2nd ed]. Boston, Little, Brown, 1986. P. 270.)

Axonal Neuropathy

Axonal neuropathy is a disorder of the neuron which causes a "dying-back" reaction of the axon. Exposure to a toxin or metabolic failure results in an inability to maintain a full length of distal membrane. Consequently, the largest neurons, those with the longest axons, are affected first. Loss of distal axon is associated with distal degeneration (Fig. 1-7). As the synapse is abandoned, there is a loss of trophic effect on muscle fibers and denervation change. Many muscle fibers are reinnervated by collateral sprouts of neighboring axons, but some are left to "wither on the vine." In severe axonal neuropathy, the result is *neurogenic atrophy* in distal muscles. Neurogenic atrophy is distinguished from atrophy of disuse, a mild condition directly related to lack of regular muscle activity. (This process is exemplified by the loss of muscle in a limb that has been cast.)

Recovery of function in axonal neuropathy is slow, and often partial. Incomplete regeneration of sensory nerves may be particularly distressing due to aberrant sensory messages (dysesthesia) and pain. Axonal neuropathy occurs with extreme B vitamin malnutrition, observed in the prisoner-of-war camps of Asia during World War II. Some veterans of the conflict emerged from long periods of internment with beriberi, a peripheral disorder due to thiamine deficiency. Among patients with severe neuropathy, some were unable to support weight or walked with a footdrop. Recovery required 6 to 18 months of good nutrition, and was occasionally incomplete.

Various experimental toxic neuropathies have been described which serve as a model for axonal neuropathy of nutritional or metabolic cause. Schaumburg and Spencer have studied the neurotoxicity of iminodiproprionitrile (IDPN), a nitrile related to the plant toxin which produces lathyrism. The substance produces a peripheral nerve disorder in animals. Tracer studies show a failure of the slow axon transport system after exposure to IDPN. The pathology shows proximal axonal swellings, with neurofilament accumulation. The distal delivery of neurofilaments is impaired, ultimately resulting in atrophy and degeneration of distal axon.

Vincristine is a plant alkaloid widely used for cancer chemotherapy. It binds microtubule proteins and interferes with cell mitosis; it disrupts neurotubules in the axon. Alterations in fast axoplasmic transport have been identified in animals treated with vincristine. One hypothesis holds that the disorder in axoplasmic transport is related to the effect of vincristine on neurotubules. Chronic exposure above a certain threshold produces a peripheral neuropathy syndrome in man. Patients complain of distal numbness and paresthesias; some loss of power and reflexes is evident in the lower extremities.

Acrylamide is a model for a third category of neuropathic toxin, producing distal axonopathy. With exposure to acrylamide there is loss of retrograde transport, which somehow impedes filament assembly. Distal swellings are observed in the axon, stuffed with giant neurofilaments. Distal axonopathy is observed with occupational exposure to some organic chemicals, such as *n*-hexane and methylethylketone. Habitual sniffers of model airplane glue can develop a chronic neuropathy from exposure to these substances.

Segmental Demyelination

A second pattern of reaction in peripheral nervous tissue is segmental demyelination. In this case, it is the Schwann cell which suffers from the effects of disease. The result is a randomly distributed loss of myelin segments. Again, the longest nerves are affected, due to a greater probability of sustaining a "hit."

How does a loss of myelin compromise peripheral nerve function? Recall that myelin decreases capacitance, limiting the diffusion of current and increasing conduction velocity. When myelin is lost, conduction velocity declines dramatically. There is also a chance that impulse conduction across the demyelinated segment may fail. In myelinated fibers, voltage-sensitive sodium channels are sparse under the myelin and concentrated at the internode. When the axon is stripped, charge diffuses out, and there is a greater probability that depolarization will not propagate across the segment. This is called *conduction block*, a likely outcome if more than one segment is compromised. In addition to slowed conduction and the risk of conduction block, several other side effects of demyelination are observed. There may be a failure of high-frequency signal transmission. Occasionally, cross talk develops between pathologically demyelinated fibers (ephaptic transmission). There is no abandonment of the synapse, and no loss of trophic effects of innervation on muscle.

Recovery is more rapid after demyelinating injury (days to weeks). Remyelination is efficient in peripheral nerve, often with smaller nodes and slightly reduced conduction velocity. In the CNS, functional recovery may begin in a few days, even in the absence of demonstrable remyelination. One proposed mechanism involves the dissemination of sodium channels along the naked axon, to restore excitability.

In the early part of the century, an acute disorder of the peripheral nervous system was described: the Guillian-Barré syndrome. The presenting feature was ascending weakness and paralysis, beginning in the legs and working its way up the spinal segments. Loss of respiratory power sometimes occurred, but the outcome was good if the patient was given assisted ventilation and good supportive care. The Guillian-Barré syndrome is an immune-mediated attack on the peripheral myelin. The disease mechanism is discussed in detail in Chapter 11. Because large, myelinated fibers are involved, loss of muscle strength in the lower limbs and loss of reflexes are early features. The weakness reaches a maximum in 2 to 3 weeks, as myelin is progressively stripped. Recovery occurs over a few months, although improvement is slow and sometimes incomplete if there is secondary axon damage.

Diabetic Neuropathy

The commonest and most important cause of peripheral nerve disease in the United States is diabetes. (In other parts of the world, leprosy is still prevalent.) In diabetic neuropathy, there is a mixed reaction, with axon loss, scattered segmental demyelination, and some vascular damage to connective tissue stroma. Teased-fiber analysis has demonstrated substantial attrition of large fibers in addition to damaged small fibers, the combination of which produces the analgesia and pain. Several clinical patterns are observed. Painful, distal symmetric sensory-motor neuropathy is the most typical. Loss of unmyelinated fibers may cause autonomic neuropathy: postural hypotension, bladder dysfunction, diarrhea, loss of cardiovascular reflexes. Nerve infarcts are occasionally described.

Entrapment Neuropathy

Single nerves may be damaged from compression or entrapment. These common ailments result from design flaws in the human anatomy, where nerves are in close proximity to the hard surface of bone or ligament. The commonest site of entrapment is the carpel ligament, located in the flexor compartment of the wrist. Compromise of the median nerve at this site, the carpel tunnel syndrome, is quite common, and easily remedied by a small surgical procedure. Other common sites of compression or entrapment are illustrated in Figure 1-1, including the ulnar nerve at the elbow, the radial nerve against the humerus ("Saturday night palsy"), and the peroneal nerve at the fibular head.

In entrapment neuropathy, there is mechanical pressure against a segment of nerve. This results in a physical squashing, and the intussusception of myelin at the internode. Destruction of the internode and segmental loss of myelin have the functional consequences reviewed above. The nerve is usually capable of good recovery once the stricture is relieved. More severe injuries involve loss of blood supply (ischemia), axon damage, and some scarring. Under these circumstances, recovery may be less satisfactory.

Causalgia

Some patients with an injury to a nerve or nerve trunk experience a continuous, severe, burning pain, which may be associated with vasomotor and trophic changes in the affected limb. Any stimulation of the skin on the affected limb (e.g., light touch) is experienced as exquisitely irritating. The painful area sometimes migrates along the limb, and does not respect nerve territory or dermatomal borders. This phenomenon, known as *causalgia,* was first described in patients suffering nerve injury in wartime. It is sometimes explained as a product of ephaptic transmission (cross talk) between sensory afferents and autonomic efferents. Pain is a prominent part of the syndrome, is diffuse and poorly localized, and does not respond well to segmental nerve block.

NERVE CONDUCTION VELOCITY

Large mixed nerves can be excited electrically, directly through the skin and subcutaneous tissues. Using a bipolar nerve stimulator, the underlying axons can be depolarized to threshold. The action potential thus evoked is conducted orthograde (and retrograde) along the nerve, and will produce a small contraction in the innervated muscle fibers. The compound muscle action potential can be recorded using surface electrodes. In this way it is then possible to stimulate and record from the limb of a cooperative patient in order to measure motor nerve conduction velocity. Provided small voltages are used, the procedure is not painful.

To record the motor conduction velocity, the median nerve is often chosen, though any large mixed nerve will do. Surface electrodes are placed over the thenar hand muscles. The nerve is stimulated at the wrist, and subsequently at a second site in the proximal arm. The time interval is measured between shock artifact and the onset of the muscle potential for both sites (Fig. 1-8). The motor nerve conduction velocity is then calculated, based on the time difference and the distance. A normal conduction velocity for the median nerve is 50 to 60 m/sec. An impulse can also be recorded from the nerve after electrical stimulation of sensory afferents. This waveform represents the sensory nerve action potential; its conduction velocity can be figured in a similar fashion.

In a demyelinating neuropathy, the nerve conduction velocity is slowed. Values under 20 m/sec are not unheard of. In a standard axonal peripheral neuropathy, the test may be unrevealing. Conduction velocity is often normal or near normal across proximal segments. Distally, there may be loss of amplitude, or failure to elicit the sensory nerve action potential. Evidence of denervation will often be apparent when the corresponding muscles are studied. In the carpel tunnel syndrome (median nerve entrapment in the wrist), the nerve conduction will likewise be normal across proximal segments. A prolonged distal latency will reflect the damage to myelin at the site of entrapment.

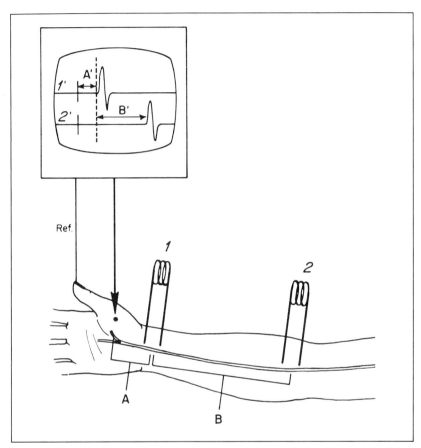

FIGURE 1-8. Measurement of motor nerve conduction velocity. The median nerve is stimulated at the wrist (1), while the compound muscle action potential is recorded from thenar hand muscles. The latency is recorded (A'). The nerve is then stimulated proximally in the forearm (2), and the latency is again recorded. The difference in latencies is calculated (B'). The conduction velocity is derived by dividing the distance traversed across the forearm (B, in meters) by the time elapsed (B', in seconds). (From R.D. Adams and M. Victor, *Principles of Neurology* [3rd ed.]. New York: McGraw-Hill, 1985, p. 955, with permission.)

REGENERATION

Peripheral nervous tissues have great capacity for regeneration and repair in response to injury. Before considering the regeneration of axons, we need first to review mechanisms for the growth of axons during development. The active area of growth at the end of the axon is the *growth cone*. Its processes move like the pseudopods of an

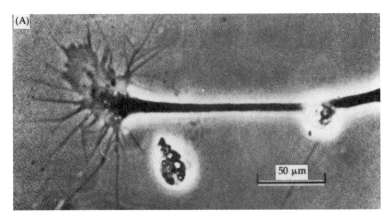

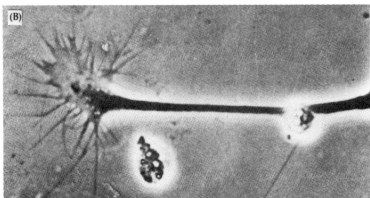

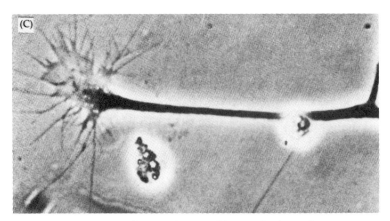

FIGURE 1-9. Pictures taken at 20-second intervals show the movements of the growth cone of a sensory neuron in tissue culture. The three frames show active changes in the filopodia. (From D. Purves and J. Lichtman, *Principles of Neural Development*. Sunderland, Mass.: Sinauer Associates, 1985, p. 97, with permission.)

amoeba, exploring the local environment (Fig. 1-9). Before the synapse is established, the growth cone is the neuron's active interface; it "recognizes," adheres to, and moves along cell surfaces. The remainder of the axon cylinder follows.

Trophic factors and cell surface molecules influence the process of axonal growth. Nerve growth factor promotes the growth of neural crest–derived tissues: cells of the dorsal root ganglia and autonomic ganglia. Motor neurons send their distal processes out into the periphery under the influence of a trophic factor as yet unidentified. The strength of adhesion to tissue planes and cell surface components are important determinants of growth in tissue culture. In the peripheral nervous system in vivo, neurites cling to adjacent axons and the basal lamina of the nerve sheath as a mechanical guide. Schwann cells also play an important role in promoting growth.

How do developing axons make appropriate synaptic connections? Specific molecular markers may be important in this process, but the details are not presently known. Initially, there is a redundant ingrowth of axons to innervate the target area. As specific connections are made during a critical period of development, some nerve processes are unsuccessful in the competition for synaptic sites. The excess neurons undergo preprogrammed cell death. During the development of the the chick embryo, for instance, there is a 30 to 50 percent loss of motor neurons as the limb bud is innervated.

Requirements for a Successful Outcome During Regeneration

When peripheral nervous tissues are injured, sprouting occurs and growth cones appear promptly at the cut end of the severed axons (Fig. 1-10). Preservation of a mechanical surface guide (the nerve sheath) and reactive Schwann cells are usually sufficient to promote regeneration. Failure to establish a pathway for regrowth sometimes results in the formation of a *neuroma*. This fatty wad of mechanically irritable nerve endings is often a source of pain. The zone of active growth in a regenerating nerve is also mechanically irritable, though generally not painful. A tap on the distal end of the growing nerve will establish and propagate sensory potentials, and the patient may report a mild electrical shock–like sensation (Tinel's sign). This test can be used to follow the progress of nerve regeneration in a limb. During reinnervation, axons make specific and appropriate synaptic connections: motor neurons to muscle fibers, sensory and autonomic fibers to the appropriate target tissue. In rare instances, errors are made. Some patients who have recovered from injury to the facial nerve, for instance, may produce tears inappropriately during facial expression.

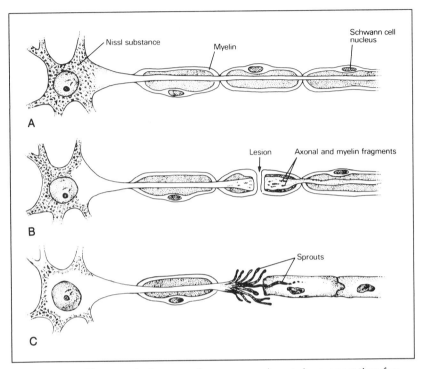

FIGURE 1-10. Changes that occur when an axon is cut, in preparation for regeneration. After 2 to 3 days, the cell body begins to swell and Nissl substance undergoes chromatolysis (see wallerian degeneration). Within a week, the proximal cut end exhibits sprouting, as new axonal growth cones are established. (From E.R. Kandel and J.H. Schwartz [eds.], *Principles of Neural Science* [2nd ed.]. New York: Elsevier, 1985, p. 191, with permission.)

In the CNS, the capacity for regeneration is quite limited. The problem lies not in the axon, but in its local environment. Regrowth of primary sensory afferents from the dorsal root ganglion stops abruptly when the nerve processes enter the spinal cord. They may be unable to get oriented or to establish a mechanical guide. Oligodendroglia may be less successful than Schwann cells at fostering axonal growth. The milieu for regeneration and repair is undoubtedly affected by the proliferation of astrocytes after injury. Under usual circumstances, regeneration is limited to 1 to 2 mm in the CNS, and is ineffective over distances. A variety of transplantation techniques are being explored to overcome this limitation. In animal studies, pieces of peripheral nerve can be engrafted as a bridge to promote regeneration over long distances within the CNS.

BIBLIOGRAPHY

Asbury, A.K., and Johnson, P.C. *Pathology of Peripheral Nerve.* Philadelphia: Saunders, 1978.

Dawson, D., Hallett, M., and Millander, L. *Entrapment Neuropathy* (2nd ed.). Boston: Little, Brown, 1990.

Katz, B. *Nerve, Muscle, and Synapse.* New York: McGraw-Hill, 1966.

Purves, D., and Lichtman, J.W. *Principles of Neural Development.* Sunderland, Mass.: Sinauer Associates, 1985.

Spencer, P., and Schaumburg, H. *Experimental and Clinical Neurotoxicology.* Baltimore: Williams & Wilkins, 1980.

Sumner, A.J. (ed.). *The Physiology of Peripheral Nerve Disease.* Philadelphia: Saunders, 1980.

Waxman, S. (ed.). *Physiology and Pathobiology of Axons.* New York: Raven Press, 1978.

CHAPTER 2

Muscle

Unless you're built like Arnold Schwarzenegger, muscle makes up roughly 35 percent of your body mass, and receives 40 percent of your cardiac output. Muscle is the only tissue in the body capable of mechanical work. It is metabolically active, and responsible for a large share of substrate utilization during physical activity. Even at rest, we rely on muscle to maintain posture and respirations.

Within a connective tissue sheath lie fascicles of individual muscle fibers. Muscle fibers are multinucleate, with nuclei lying along the basal lamina. The external membrane is highly trabeculated. A specialized region, the motor end plate receives the synapse for each muscle fiber. The muscle spindle, a thin fiber bundle with stretch receptors, is arranged in parallel with the working fibers of the muscle. It is a specialized structure, which provides sensory feedback essential for the regulation of muscle tone. Spindle fibers are of two types: nuclear bag fibers and nuclear chain fibers. The nonspindle muscle fibers are sometimes designated as "extrafusal," a terminology almost certain to confuse.

Muscle fibers contain excitable membrane, a variety of cytoskeleton proteins, and myofibrils. Myofibrils are the working unit of contraction. They make up 75 percent of the tissue. The myofibril is divided into segments (sarcomeres), each a linear array of contractile proteins (Fig. 2-1). The thick filaments contain myosin proteins; the thin filaments contain actin, troponin, and tropomyosin. The sliding, linear arrangement of contractile elements gives the sarcomere a banded appearance. The myofibril is surrounded by a network of sarcoplasmic reticulum (SR). Circumferentially run an array of T tubules, apposed on either side by SR to form a triad. The T system acts to release calcium during depolarization of the muscle fiber, and sequester calcium when the fiber is quiet.

When acetylcholine is released at the neuromuscular junction, the muscle fiber responds by shortening to produce a mechanical force. This event can be viewed as having three steps: (1) electrical excitation

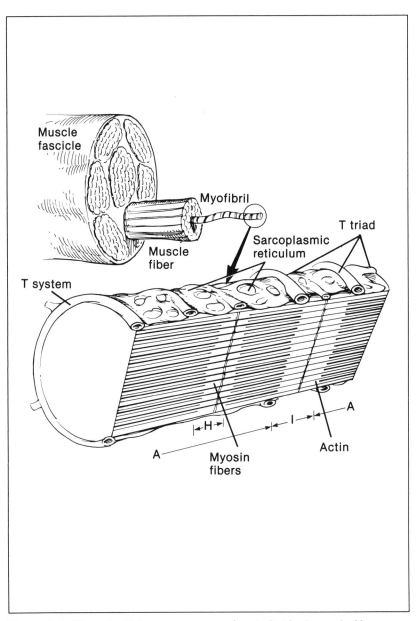

FIGURE 2-1. The subcellular components of an individual muscle fiber (myofibril). The linear arrangement of actin and myosin proteins produces a banded appearance. A sarcomere is the unit between Z lines. Each sarcomere contains two T tubule triads. (Modified from   C.M. Pearson and F.K. Mostofi [eds.], *The Striated Muscle.* Baltimore: Williams & Wilkins, 1974, with permission.)

of the muscle fiber, (2) excitation-contraction coupling, and (3) the interaction of muscle proteins to produce shortening. The muscle membrane is susceptible to the same ionic forces that depolarize the axon. There are more voltage-gated calcium channels in muscle membrane, compared to nerve. Consequently the muscle fiber can be fired even when the sodium channels are inactivated (e.g., by tetrodotoxin). Postsynaptic potentials at the neuromuscular junction are adequate to produce an action potential, which propagates along the muscle fiber.

Calcium is the internal signal which couples the electrical event to muscle contraction. There is normally a gradient (about 1,000 : 1) between extracellular calcium and the free concentration inside the muscle fiber. Depolarization of the membrane activates the T system, which releases calcium from the SR into the myofibril. Within the sarcomere, calcium promotes the contractile process. An active mechanism sequesters calcium into the SR when the cell is repolarized. Calcium-adenosine triphosphatase (ATPase) promotes the reuptake of calcium, allowing the muscle fiber to "relax."

Contraction is produced by the interaction of actin with myosin S1 protein. The sliding filament model shows how these proteins are apposed (Fig. 2-2). A chemical reaction causes the actin filament to "crawl" along the myosin 10 nm, which consumes adenosine triphosphate (ATP) and shortens the myofibril. The interaction is blocked by tropomyosin in the normal (inactive) configuration of the muscle. When calcium is released, it binds troponin protein and causes a confirmational shift. Tropomyosin is displaced from the active site, and the actin and myosin interact as described. The process is reversed (the reaction goes downhill) when calcium is removed. After death, there is inadequate ATP to pump away calcium and release contraction, and *rigor mortis* sets in.

ENERGY METABOLISM

Because muscles do all the mechanical work, they require extensive metabolic support. Energy metabolism to drive skeletal muscle consumes a large proportion of the body's available substrate resources. The high metabolic rate of working muscle renders it vulnerable to a variety of metabolic disorders.

The contractile process and the calcium pump consume ATP. High-energy phosphate in the form of ATP is the proximate source of energy for skeletal muscle. The reserves of ATP are quite limited. Much of the energy readily available to muscle is stored in the form of phosphocreatine. Creatine phosphokinase (CK) catalyzes the formation of

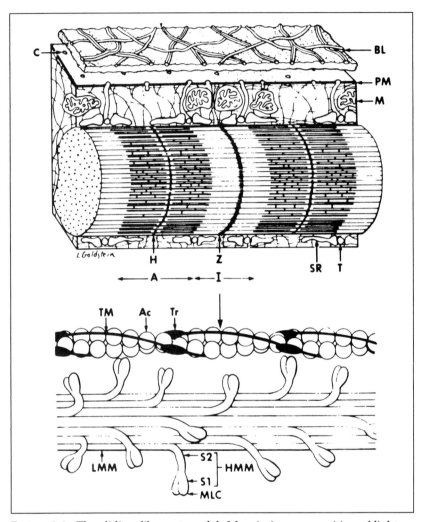

Figure 2-2. The sliding filament model. Myosin is a composition of light (LMM) and heavy (HMM) meromyosin. The actin filament (Ac) slides along the myosin protein during contraction. Tropomyosin (TM) inhibits the reaction, until a conformational change is induced by calcium. BL = basal lamina; M = mitochondria; PM = plasma membrane; SR = sarcoplasmic reticulum; T = T tubule. (From A.K. Asbury, G.M. McKhann, and W.I. McDonald, *Diseases of the Nervous System.* Philadelphia: Saunders, 1986, p. 191, with permission.)

Figure 2-3. Anaerobic metabolism of carbohydrate in skeletal muscle. Glucose is stored in muscle as glycogen. Glycogen is metabolized to pyruvate and lactate. Enzymatic defects known to affect man are marked with an asterisk. (Modified from S. Di Mauro, N. Bresolin, and A. Papadimitriou, Fuels for exercise. In G. Serratrice et al. [eds.], *Neuromuscular Diseases.* New York: Raven, 1984.

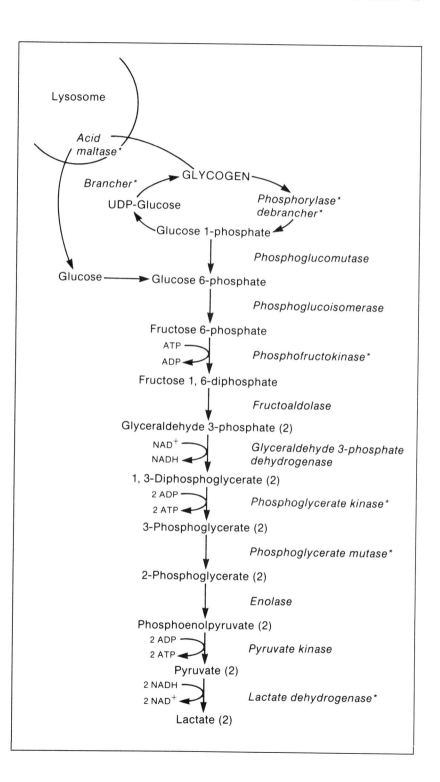

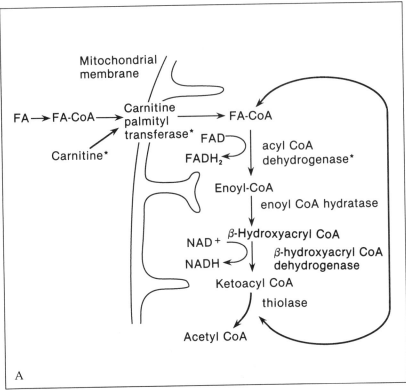

FIGURE 2-4. Metabolism (beta oxidation) of fatty acids (FA) in skeletal muscle (A). Known metabolic defects are marked with an asterisk. Within the mitochondria, acyl–coenzyme A (CoA) and Krebs cycle metabolites are oxidized fully, using the electron transfer system (B). Patients with blocks of the respiratory chain affecting complex I or complex III may exhibit exercise intolerance. (From A.K. Asbury, G.M. McKhann, and W.I. McDonald, *Diseases of the Nervous System.* Philadelphia: Saunders, 1986, p. 245, with permission.)

ATP from phosphocreatine. Large quantities of CK are found in muscle tissue. Creatine phosphokinase occasionally leaks out of muscle membrane and into the circulation in the presence of muscle damage or disease.

To restore high-energy phosphate, muscle has two options: metabolism of carbohydrate or fatty acid. Glycogen is available to muscle as a stored source of carbohydrate. Figure 2-3 summarizes the events of glycogen metabolism under anaerobic conditions. There is enough glycogen stored to work intensively for 3 to 4 hours, often long enough to help run a marathon or put in a half day of tough physical labor. This kind of work is hard, and lactate makes the muscles burn.

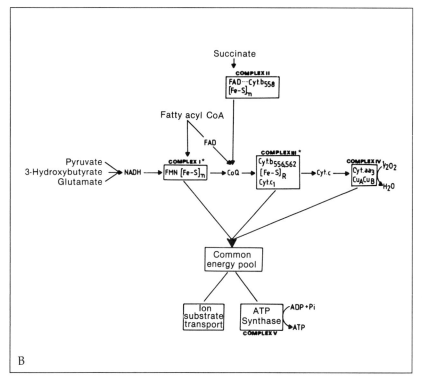

FIGURE 2-4 (Continued).

Oxidative metabolism of fatty acids is a more efficient energy source for slow steady jobs. The pathway for fatty acid metabolism is summarized in Figure 2-4. The main events transpire inside mitochondria, which are scattered about the muscle fiber. Carnitine is the carrier which accompanies fatty acids into the mitochondria. Ultimately the electron transfer system is utilized to couple the production of NADH with the regeneration of ATP.

How the two energy sources are used depends on the intensity and duration of exertion. At rest, muscles utilize fatty acid oxidation as an energy source. To generate peak power for brief periods (high-intensity exercise), carbohydrate is burned under largely anaerobic conditions. In more moderate exercise, the choice of substrate depends on the duration of work. Glycogen is used initially, supplemented by blood glucose. With continuing exertion, fatty acid metabolism becomes a more important source. Approaching 4 hours, as glycogen stores are expended, lipid is the principal fuel, supplemented by some catabolism of amino acids.

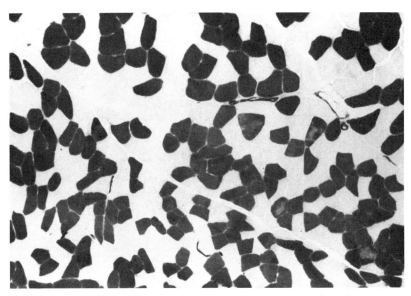

FIGURE 2-5. Normal muscle biopsy, frozen section stained for adenosine triphosphatase. At pH 9.4, type II fibers are preferentially stained. A normal checkerboard pattern of type I and type II fibers is observed. (From Dr. James Morris, Brigham and Womens Hospital, Boston.)

Muscle fibers are specialized for a particular task. Type I fibers contain abundant mitochondria, and prefer oxidative metabolism. These fibers are slower in response, and more fatigue-resistant. They do long steady work. An abundance of type I fibers, rich in mitochondrial enzymes, gives the appearance of dark meat to the leg muscles of a turkey. Type II fibers, by contrast, are specialized for glycolysis. They are fast in response, and develop a brief burst of peak power. A preponderance of type II fibers with abundant glycogen stores provides the appearance of white meat to the breast muscles. Type II fibers become burdened with lactate during peak exertion, and tend to fatigue. Type I and type II fibers exist together in mammalian skeletal muscle, in an average ratio of 1 : 2. They can be differentiated in fresh tissue from muscle biopsy by histochemical stains. ATPase at pH 9.4 preferentially stains type II fibers, which can be observed in cross section in skeletal muscle in Figure 2-5.

SYNDROMES OF MUSCLE DISEASE

Disease of skeletal muscle can present in a limited number of ways. Both acute and chronic muscle disorders are observed. Many defects of skeletal muscle are present from birth. In the muscular dystrophies, there is a progressive loss of function as the programmed genetic defect is expressed.

Figure 2-6 provides an approach to the diseases of skeletal muscle. Three principal syndromes are described. Most often, muscle disease presents with *progressive proximal weakness*. Palpable loss of muscle bulk and change in posture are associated features. Onset is insidious and gradual, as observed with the muscular dystrophies, congenital and metabolic myopathies. Inflammatory diseases of muscle are more often acute or subacute, and may be associated with muscle edema or pain.

A second presentation is episodic failure, related to exertion. This syndrome is observed with disorders of substrate utilization. *Exercise intolerance and cramps* are the principal symptoms. There may be lysis of muscle fibers with release of myoglobin into the circulation (and myoglobinuria). Myophosphorylase deficiency (McArdle's disease) exemplifies this pattern of clinical expression. A third list of diseases is associated with a specific *failure of the contractile process*. Myotonia and myotonic dystrophy will be reviewed in more detail; myasthenia gravis is discussed in Chapters 3 and 11.

Space does not permit a discussion of all the common disorders, let alone the rare inborn errors of metabolism. A disease from each category is presented, in order to examine some of the issues relating to expression of muscle pathology.

Muscular Dystrophy

The dystrophies are genetically determined disorders, characterized by progressive degeneration of skeletal muscle. Most of these diseases are slowly progressive; some are compatible with a normal life expectancy. They are selective, and not all muscles are affected by each disease. The hallmark of a dystrophic disorder is segmental muscle fiber necrosis and replacement of muscle by fibrous tissue, resulting in progressive weakness.

The most tragic and severe muscle disease is Duchenne's dystrophy. This fatal disorder has its onset in early childhood, and produces progressive incapacity. Affected individuals are in a wheelchair by 7 to 12 years of age, and death usually occurs in the early twenties. The disease follows an X-linked pattern of inheritance, and is primarily observed in boys. Normal in appearance at birth, affected individuals are slow to walk. When they learn, a waddling gait is observed due to weakness of the proximal pelvic muscles, and the abdomen protrudes. Calf muscles are weak, but have *pseudohypertrophy* (fatty enlargement). Proximal weakness is most evident when patients try to get up from the floor. Serum CK is strikingly elevated.

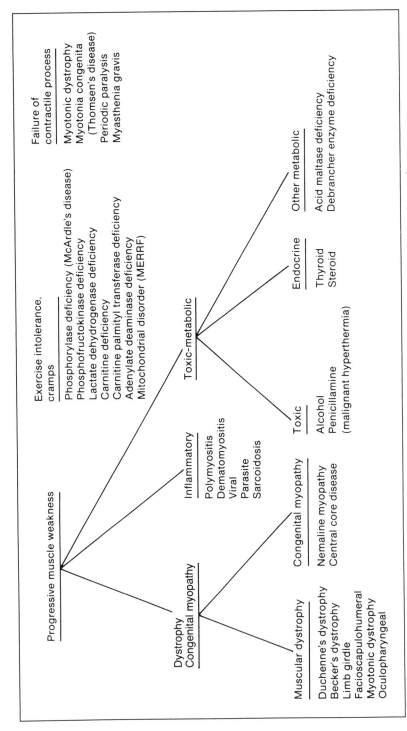

FIGURE 2-6. Disorders of muscle: An organizing approach to the common disorders of skeletal muscle.

The genetic defect has been localized to the short arm of the X chromosome. Spontaneous mutations occur relatively commonly (unlike the situation in Huntington's disease). The gene abnormality has been identified through linkage studies, and its product has been synthesized in the laboratory by Kunkel and associates. The protein dystrophin is absent in Duchenne's dystrophy patients. It has some homology to the actin protein, and is found in association with the T system. A working hypothesis suggests that impaired sequestration of calcium leads to membrane damage, leakage of CK out of the muscle fiber, and ultimately to segmental necrosis of muscle. Researchers are now looking for a way to replace the missing constituent of muscle fibers in affected patients.

Polymyositis

The term *myositis* refers to an active inflammatory disease of muscle. Several microorganisms are known to infect muscle, including influenza viruses, coxsackievirus, *Staphylococcus aureus*, *Toxoplasma*, and trichinae, the etiologic agent of trichinosis, a parasite infection contracted from eating undercooked pork. Many cases of myositis are idiopathic inflammatory disorders, connective tissue diseases, the most important being polymyositis.

Polymyositis is a manifestation of autoimmunity, an attack by the body's immune system on its own muscles. The presentation is sometimes acute, with fever, muscle ache, and systemic symptoms. More often, onset is gradual over weeks or months. Patients have diffuse proximal weakness, sometimes manifest as difficulty climbing stairs or getting out of a chair. Involved muscles may be painful. The condition is called *dermatomyositis* when skin changes occur in association. Sometimes other features of connective tissue disease are associated; 5 to 15 percent of patients have systemic lupus erythematosus, rheumatoid arthritis, or scleroderma. There is segmental necrosis of muscle, with an inflammatory, mononuclear cell infiltrate. The exact mechanism of immune attack on muscle has not been defined; autoantibodies may play a role. Treatment is generally directed at immunosuppression, using steroids and/or cytotoxic drugs.

Endocrine Myopathy

Hormones that affect intermediary metabolism have a direct impact on skeletal muscle. Disorders of the thyroid and changes in steroid hormones produce manifestations in muscle. Hyperthyroidism causes mild, diffuse muscular weakness in a majority of patients, and is infrequently so severe as to be a presenting complaint. Some thyrotoxic patients have periodic paralysis. Hypothyroidism has a more serious impact on muscle. Stretch reflexes have delayed relaxation, and serum CK is elevated. Myalgia and muscle stiffness are common complaints.

A common metabolic myopathy in general practice results from the use of corticosteroids. (A similar pattern may be observed in Cushing's syndrome.) High-dose, daily administration of steroids over months can produce a proximally distributed myopathy. The proximal leg muscles are most involved; they become small and fatty. Serum CK is normal. Exogenous administration of androgens, on the other hand, causes gross muscle hypertrophy and supranormal strength. Professional athletes have been known to abuse hormones, though the National Collegiate Athletic Association and the Olympic committee frown on the practice.

McArdle's Disease: A Disorder of Substrate Utilization

Inborn errors of metabolism affect energy production in muscle. Many of these disorders are symptomatic during exercise. Patients may appear fully strong at rest, but develop cramps and muscle ache during exertion. Failure to keep up with metabolic demand during vigorous exercise can result in fiber damage and myoglobinuria. This presentation is seen particularly with disorders of carbohydrate utilization, but also with defects involving fatty acid or mitochondrial metabolism. Carbohydrate defects are more dramatic, as they impair delivery of peak power during maximal effort.

Muscle phosphorylase deficiency (McArdle's disease) is one of the glycogen storage diseases. Symptoms begin during adolescence or early adult life. Patients present with painful muscle cramps during exercise. The disease sometimes goes unrecognized, as symptoms seem functional in nature and patients appear normal between attacks. Severe attacks liberate CK and myoglobin from muscle fibers; myoglobinuria may be large enough to cause renal failure.

The enzyme deficiency is inherited in an autosomal recessive pattern. Excess glycogen storage can be appreciated on muscle biopsy. Measurement of lactate during forearm exercise is a useful diagnostic test. This is done with a tourniquet, in order to produce ischemic (anaerobic) conditions. Failure to elaborate lactate is characteristic of defects in carbohydrate utilization.

Myotonia: Myotonic Dystrophy

Myotonia is an abnormality in the electrical activity of muscle fibers, resulting in excess irritability and sustained contraction. Involuntary contraction is observed following mechanical stimulation, and there is a failure to relax after full voluntary contraction. The phenomenon is observed in a variety of disorders, but most commonly in myotonic dystrophy.

Myotonic dystrophy is an inherited disorder, somewhat variable in severity. It usually presents in adult life. There is slowly progressive weakness of proximal muscle, and a variable degree of myotonia. Other traits make the disease distinctive and recognizable. Atrophy of the temporalis and masseter muscles gives a "hatchet-faced" appearance. Male patients have frontal balding and testicular atrophy. Other associated features include endocrine disturbances and cataracts. Patients experience difficulty relaxing their handgrip. Myotonia can be elicited by percussion of the thenar hand muscles. Insertion of electromyographic (EMG) needle electrodes is associated with a characteristic manifestation of irritability: crescendo-decrescendo potentials which, when amplified, sound like a dive bomber, or the revving of a small engine.

The disorder is autosomal dominant in inheritance, with the locus on chromosome 19. The mechanism for the myotonia is not well understood. In an animal model, the myotonic sheep, there is a disorder of the membrane chloride channel. Decreased ion current through the chloride channel enhances irritability and alters the course of repolarization. A similar phenomenon can be induced pharmacologically with 20,23-diazocholesterol. In human myotonic dystrophy, the abnormality probably lies elsewhere, in the voltage-gated sodium or potassium channel. As it becomes possible to administer drugs which modify the actions of single ion channels, better understanding of the mechanism and even treatment may be possible.

DISORDERS OF THE MOTOR NEURON

The motor unit is the effector for the vertebrate nervous system. It transforms electrical signals from the brain and spinal cord into mechanical forces. The act of muscle contraction which enables voluntary movement depends entirely on the recruitment of the appropriate set of motor units.

The motor unit consists of the motor neuron, its axon, terminal branches, and those muscle fibers in a skeletal muscle which it specifically innervates (Fig. 2-7). The cell body of the motor neuron resides in the anterior gray matter of the spinal cord (or motor cranial nerve nucleus), where it receives numerous synaptic inputs from spinal interneurons and upper motor neurons. Its axon exits in the ventral root of the segmental nerve and travels in the peripheral nervous system within a mixed nerve. Its destination lies in the belly of one of

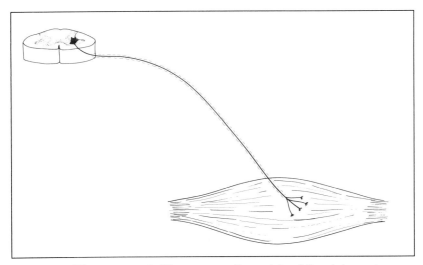

Figure 2-7. The motor unit: The motor unit consists of the alpha motor neuron in the anterior gray of the spinal cord, its axon and terminal branches, and all the muscle fibers it specifically innervates.

over 600 skeletal muscles. The terminal branches make synapses with individual muscle fibers at a specialized region known as the motor end plate.

Thousands of motor units populate each muscle. They vary in size: a single motor unit may include up to 300 muscle fibers. Units from a small muscle, such as an extraocular muscle, which is specialized for precision, may contain only a few muscle fibers (a low *innervation ratio*). Units from a large muscle like the quadriceps, which is specialized for power, are large and crude and have numerous big muscle fibers (a high innervation ratio).

Patients with disease of the motor unit present with muscular atrophy and weakness. When considering nervous system disorders that cause weakness, it is traditional to separate lower motor neuron disorders from those affecting the various upper motor neuron pathways. The anterior horn cell (lower motor neuron) is vulnerable because it supports a large axon. There is a limited population of such nerve cells, which are essential for movement, and they cannot be replaced when they are lost. Consequently, disease of these neurons produces a dramatic and often irreversible clinical syndrome.

The *lower motor neuron syndrome* is characterized by weakness, muscle atrophy, motor unit irritability, and a decrease in muscle tone and stretch reflexes. Weakness and atrophy occur from loss of motor units, which reduces the capacity of the muscle to do work. Atrophy can occur with disuse also, but when motor units are lost the reduction in power is much greater. Several changes occur in the motor unit as a result of a denervating disease. Individual muscle fibers in sick units become hyperirritable and fire spontaneously. This spontaneous activity of single fibers is known as *fibrillation*. Whole units can also display spontaneous activity. This produces a visible muscle twitch, a *fasciculation*. Fibrillations and fasciculations begin 10 to 14 days after motor neuron injury; fasciculations persist as long as the injured motor neurons remain excitable. With chronic denervation of muscle, a reorganization occurs in the innervation pattern (Fig. 2-8). Vacant denervated fibers are often taken over by adjacent units. This reinnervation results in a smaller number of oversized, often giant, units. The fine control over muscle power is diminished. These units produce coarse fasciculations when distressed. As a large number of motor units are lost, there is a corresponding reduction in muscle tone (flaccid paralysis) and decreased amplitude in the stretch reflex.

Amyotrophic Lateral Sclerosis

Amyotrophic lateral sclerosis (ALS) is a disease of both upper and lower motor neurons; denervation atrophy of muscle (amyotrophy) is usually a prominent finding. Variants occur, in which the presentation involves limb muscles (progressive muscular atrophy) or cranial muscles (progressive bulbar palsy). Onset usually occurs in the fifties or sixties. The loss of motor units is progressive and debilitating, resulting in death from respiratory failure or pneumonia within 5 years.

The disease spares extraocular muscles, small muscles with a low innervation ratio. It also spares autonomic innervation of smooth muscles (the bladder, bowel, and sphincters). Sensory systems and CNS cholinergic neurons are also spared, indicating *selective vulnerability* of the motor system. It is unclear what makes the motor neuron vulnerable. The answer may lie in a surface marker, or perhaps some special metabolic function. The mechanism of injury is unknown.

Poliomyelitis

Polio is an acute viral infection of the motor neuron. It was an epidemic illness in the 1950s. Once a major public health problem, polio was virtually eradicated by a successful vaccination program in the United States. Acute paralytic polio is an infection of the anterior horn cell. As motor units are lost, patients have pain, cramps, and evolution

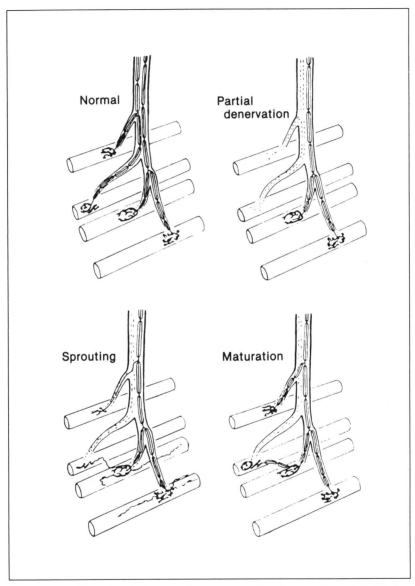

FIGURE 2-8. Alteration in innervation pattern after denervation of skeletal muscle. After injury to a motor nerve, severed axons degenerate. Within days, sprouts emerge from intact nerve endings and nodes. These regenerating processes seek out end plates on denervated muscle fibers. One to two months later, sprouts innervating end plates are retained, while unsuccessful sprouts disappear. Such giant units are typical of neurogenic atrophy. (From M.C. Brown, R.L. Holland, and W.G. Hopkins, Motor nerve sprouting. Reproduced, with permission, from the *Annual Review of Neuroscience*, Vol. 4, © 1981 by Annual Reviews Inc.)

of the lower motor neuron syndrome. Involvement of respiratory muscles is (was) common, requiring ventilator support. Some recovery occurs from reinnervation and repair of damaged units. Many motor units are killed altogether by the virus, and most patients have residual muscle atrophy.

A curious problem was described more recently in survivors of the polio epidemic. Many of these patients are now in their forties or older. Some experience in later life a slowly progressive weakness in previously affected muscles. This phenomenon is known as *postpolio syndrome*, and is an interesting and controversial entity. Some experts speculate that late loss of motor units represents an inflammatory change, a recrudescence (or persistence) of viral infection. Another hypothesis maintains that these patients have an acceleration in the normal, age-related attrition of the motor unit pool. The giant motor units that remain in affected muscle may be vulnerable due to their large size and the metabolic and synthetic activity necessary to support this size. This population of motor units may experience "early burn-out" and accelerated cell death. To date, there has been no evidence of persistent infection, and recent studies favor this latter hypothesis.

LABORATORY INVESTIGATION OF MUSCLE DISEASE: EMG AND MUSCLE BIOPSY

Electromyography is a technique for examining the electrical activity of skeletal muscle. As an extension of the physical examination, it is a very useful procedure in the diagnosis of neuromuscular disease. It is particularly helpful in separating denervation change from primary muscle disease. As the procedure is usually done, a concentric needle electrode is inserted into the muscle to record selectively the activity of individual motor units. The needle shaft acts as the indifferent electrode. It is possible to tune in a few muscle fibers near the beveled end of the needle, those fibers in close proximity to the recording electrode. Fibers in the neighborhood of the electrode belong to one of several surrounding motor units. A potential is recorded when one of the units fires and its respective muscle fibers depolarize.

Figure 2-9,A, shows the response recorded as the action potential propagates along a single muscle fiber. (A moving dipole would produce this picture as it passed by the electrode.) When an entire motor unit fires in a synchronized manner, the individual fiber potentials are superimposed to form the motor unit potential. The characteristic configuration is 5 to 15 msec in duration, and may include three or four phase reversals (Fig. 2-9,B). Needle penetration may stir up some activity, from the mechanical irritation and injury of muscle fibers.

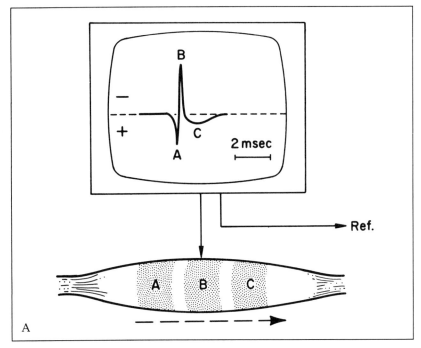

FIGURE 2-9. Normal motor unit potential. As the wave of depolarization propagates along an individual muscle fiber, the electrode "sees" a triphasic potential (A). Superimposition of all the potentials from individual muscle fibers activated by the motor neuron produces the individual motor unit potential. (From R.D. Adams and M. Victor, *Principles of Neurology* [3rd ed.]. New York: McGraw-Hill, 1985, p. 949, with permission.) B is a recording of a typical motor unit from a normal subject. The scale is indicated by the insert. The unit is roughly 6 msec in duration, and has a normal configuration. (Motor unit courtesy of Dr. Leo Davies, Spinal Cord Injury Service, Brockton/West Roxbury Veterans Administration Medical Center, Boston.)

Once this insertional activity subsides, the normal muscle is quiet at rest. As the muscle begins to contract with weak effort, smaller units are recruited first. Three or four different units may be identified, firing repetitively at rates of 5 to 10 per second. With maximal effort, a barrage of potentials of varying size can be observed, a wall of electrical activity known as the *full interference pattern*.

Abnormal EMG

While a major clinical use of EMG is to separate denervation from primary muscle disease, other kinds of abnormality can be observed. Myotonic dystrophy is associated with abnormal insertional activity.

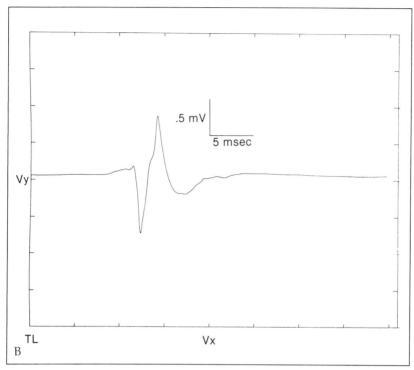

.5 mV

5 msec

Vy

TL

Vx

B

FIGURE 2-9 (Continued).

The mechanical stimulus of needle insertion provokes a storm of electrical activity, which waxes and wanes audibly over the recording amplifier. These "dive bomber potentials" are indicative of a myotonic disorder. In McArdle's disease, ischemic exercise can produce muscle contracture as energy metabolism falls behind. Muscle contracture is electrically silent, as the muscle fibers are unable to relax.

With active denervation of muscle, abnormal activity can be observed at rest. These changes begin as early as 10 to 14 days after injury. Fibrillations occur, due to the spontaneous firing of muscle fibers at rest. Fasciculations can also be recorded from resting muscle in patients with denervating disease. Chronic denervation is characterized by the appearance of giant polyphasic reinnervation units. Reinnervation units are large in amplitude because they contain extra muscle fibers. Large size of the unit within the muscle results in temporal dispersion of the potential, which is often greater than 15 msec in duration and grossly multiphasic due to late components (Fig. 2-10). At full effort, the interference pattern may be sparse due to dropout of motor units.

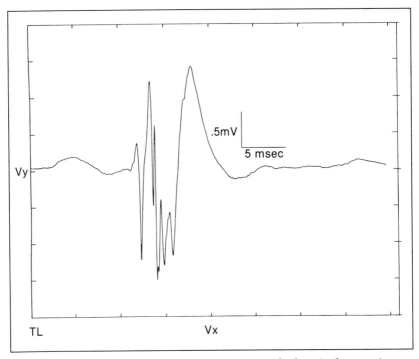

FIGURE 2-10. Giant polyphasic motor unit seen with chronic denervation. This unit is from the biceps muscle of a patient with a history of spinal cord injury. The scale is comparable to Figure 2-9, B. Units approach 2,500 μV in size, and are multiphasic. (Courtesy of Dr. Leo Davies, Spinal Cord Injury Service, Brockton/West Roxbury Veterans Administration Medical Center, Boston.)

In primary muscle disease, there is scattered segmental necrosis of muscle fibers. This results in units with diminished voltage, and fragmentation of the muscle potential (Fig. 2-11). These brief, small-amplitude polyphasic units (BSAPs) characterize the picture of primary myopathy. Fibrillations are also seen from free fragments of muscle fiber in actively destructive disorders like polymyositis. These EMG patterns are observed in a variety of primary muscle diseases, and are not specifically diagnostic.

Muscle Biopsy

When muscle disease has been identified by clinical and EMG criteria, muscle biopsy is the definitive diagnostic procedure. A variety of histochemical stains are done on fixed and fresh frozen tissue. The distinction between type I (oxidative) and type II (fast-twitch) fibers can

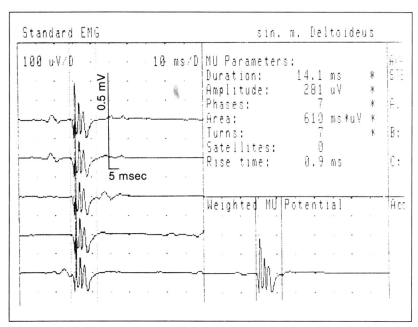

FIGURE 2-11. Motor units from a patient with myopathy. Units are small in amplitude, fragmented, and polyphasic. (From Dr. Frisso Potts, Brigham and Womens Hospital, Boston.)

be appreciated on staining for NADH or ATPase. The ATPase reaction stains type I fibers dark when done at pH 4.6; the pattern is reversed when the reaction is incubated at pH 9.4. The mixed pattern of type I and type II fibers in a cross section of normal skeletal muscle is shown in Figure 2-5.

In atrophy due to disuse, the overall arrangement of fibers is maintained, but individual muscle fibers lose mass. When atrophy is due to a chronic denervating disease, involvement is highly selective. Fibers from some of the individual motor units show denervation changes, and the checkerboard pattern of type I and type II fibers is altered by reinnervation. Innervation determines the character (histochemical type) of muscle fibers. As muscle fibers are reorganized into large units by ongoing denervation and reinnervation, fiber type grouping is evident (Fig. 2-12). Grouped atrophy is the hallmark of chronic denervating disease.

In the muscular dystrophies, characteristic changes are found on biopsy of involved muscle. There is variation in fiber size, and degeneration of some fibers. An increase is observed in connective tissue elements. No inflammatory cells are present. In polymyositis, on the other hand, active inflammatory infiltrate is found amid involved

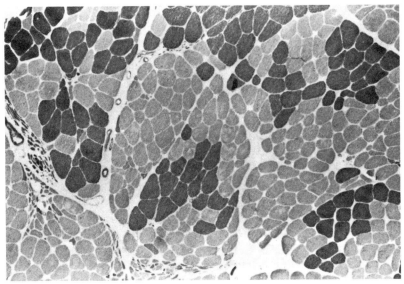

FIGURE 2-12. Muscle biopsy, stained with adenosine triphosphatase pH 9.4, taken from a patient with neurogenic atrophy. Note the clustering of type I and type II fibers. (Compare with Fig. 2-5.) Fiber-type grouping is indicative of denervation and reinnervation. (From J. Daube et al., *Medical Neurosciences* [2nd ed.]. Boston: Little, Brown, 1986. P. 284.)

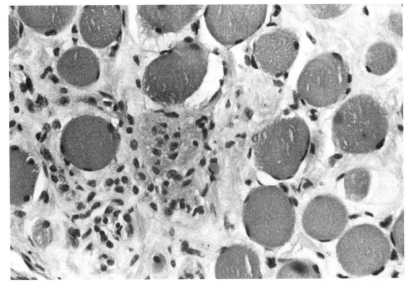

FIGURE 2-13. Muscle biopsy from patient with Duchenne's muscular dystrophy, stained with hematoxylin and eosin. There is marked variation in fiber size. Some fibers are undergoing necrosis. Connective tissue is increased. (Courtesy of Dr. Anna Sotrel, Beth Israel Hospital, Boston.)

TABLE 2-1. Summary Diagram: Neuromuscular Diseases

	Neuropathy	*Myopathy*	*Motor Neuron Disease*
Weakness	Distal	Proximal	Regional
Sensory loss	Yes	No	No
Reflex	Absent	Diminished	Variably decreased, may be increased
Atrophy	May be	Some	Pronounced
Fasciculations	Sometimes	No	Yes
EMG	Denervation changes with axonal type	BSAPs	Denervation changes, giant units
Biopsy	Grouped atrophy in axonal type	Variation in fiber size; damaged fibers, inflammatory and connective tissue	Grouped atrophy

muscle fibers (Fig. 2-13). Changes are sometimes peripherally distributed or perivascular in the muscle fascicle. In trichinosis and in toxoplasmosis, the etiologic agent, a microorganism, can be found in the muscle biopsy.

Glycogen storage or lipid accumulation can be seen in some of the metabolic disorders. Patients with mitochondrial disorders have "ragged red fibers" when stained with the Gomori trichrome method. Other pathognomonic findings identify nemaline myopathy, central core disease, sarcoidosis, and markers of the various connective tissue disorders.

The procedure is thus very useful, but care is required in the planning and harvesting of muscle biopsy to obtain optimal results. The pathologist should be involved in planning the procedure, so that appropriate stains can be performed. Table 2-1 reviews the principal categories of neuromuscular disease that can be distinguished clinically, together with their EMG and biopsy findings.

BIBLIOGRAPHY

Dubowitz, V., and Brook, M.H. *Muscle Biopsy: A Modern Approach.* London: Saunders, 1973.

Katz, B. *Nerve, Muscle, and Synapse.* New York: McGraw-Hill, 1966.

Walton, J.N. *Disorders of Voluntary Muscle.* Edinburgh: Churchill Livingston, 1974.

CHAPTER 3

Synapse: The Neuromuscular Junction

The synapse is the zone of contact across which nerve cells communicate. Within the central nervous system (CNS), neurons establish synapses with hundreds, even thousands, of other nerve cells. Both electrical and chemical synapses are described, but the chemical type predominates in the large synaptic networks of the mammalian forebrain. At the chemical synapse, depolarization of the nerve terminal causes the release of chemical messenger molecules into the synaptic cleft (Fig. 3-1). The arrival of these molecules at specialized receptor sites results in an ion current, and a transient change in the postsynaptic membrane potential. The postsynaptic neuron (or muscle cell) may reach threshold and generate its own action potential. The sum of excitatory and inhibitory postsynaptic potentials at any moment in time determines the response.

Why do nerve cells communicate in this peculiar way? There are many disadvantages. The process is slow; 10 to 20 msec can be consumed by the release of the neurotransmitter, its diffusion across the synaptic cleft, and the postsynaptic interaction. While this seems like a small amount of time, it is substantial when compared with the information handling speed of a silicon microprocessor. The neuron must be equipped for the containment and disposal of potent neuroactive micromolecules. In this arrangement, there is the potential for malfunction, mischief, and disease. Nervous tissues are vulnerable to numerous drugs and toxins that affect synaptic function.

On the positive side, chemical transmission allows for a great diversity of synaptic interactions. Messenger molecules are used of widely differing temporal persistence. Amino acid neurotransmitters such as glutamate, aspartate, and γ-aminobutyric acid (GABA) have a brief duration of synaptic effect, measured in a few milliseconds (the blink of an ion channel). Monoamines may be present slightly longer, and commonly act through a second messenger (cyclic adenosine monophosphate [cAMP] or phosphoinositide). The hydrolysis and removal of peptides may take seconds or even minutes. Likewise, the space of

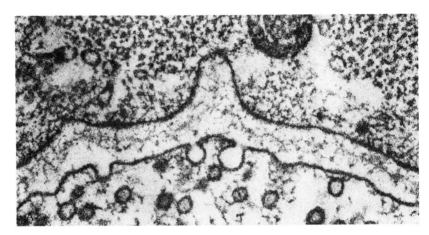

FIGURE 3-1. A. The electron micrograph shows vesicles caught in the act of discharging their contents into the frog neuromuscular junction. (From C.F. Stevens. The neuron. *Sci. Am.* 241 : 24, 1979, with permission.) B. Neurotransmitter is released into the synapse by the exocytosis of synaptic vesicles. Vesicles open as they fuse with the presynaptic membrane, a process which is illustrated schematically in the figure. (Courtesy of Dr. John E. Heuser.)

transmitter distribution may be an important variable. In the striatum, dopamine is sometimes released in nonclassic synapses, suffusing the neurons in the neighborhood. In the infundibulum and pituitary, peptides are secreted into a regional circulation. The diversity of transmitter mechanisms is a very useful feature in systems design. Another advantage of the chemical synapse is its plasticity: the synapse is a modifiable structure, which can reflect the history of previous synaptic events. It can be modulated up or down.

THE NEUROMUSCULAR JUNCTION AS AN EXAMPLE OF A CHEMICAL SYNAPSE

The synapse at the neuromuscular junction is particularly well known through the work of Fatt and Katz and others in the 1950s. As an experimental preparation, it is relatively easy to handle and study. Muscle cells are large and accessible; their innervation can be identified. Individual muscle fibers are easily penetrated by an intracellular recording electrode. The preparation can also be visualized well through interference microscopy. More recently, using patch clamp techniques, the behavior of a single postsynaptic receptor and its ion channel have been characterized.

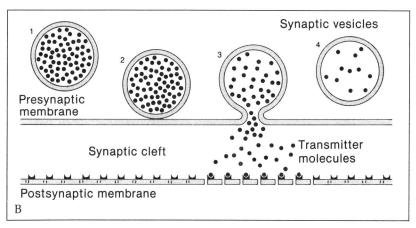

FIGURE 3-1 (Continued).

The neuromuscular junction is a special case, and has properties not typical of other chemical synapses. The target is a muscle cell and not another neuron. The synapse occurs at a specialized zone known as the *motor end plate* (Fig. 3-2). Each muscle fiber receives innervation from only one motor unit. There is no convergence of synaptic inputs. Consequently, the synapses that occur onto muscle cells are all excitatory. They are rapid, and uniquely effective. In the CNS, a typical excitatory postsynaptic potential (EPSP) achieves 1 to 5 mV in amplitude. At the neuromuscular junction, postsynaptic potentials average 60 mV, sufficient in size to exceed threshold and compel firing of the muscle action potential.

Figure 3-3 shows some of the anatomic specializations of the neuromuscular junction. At the presynaptic nerve terminal, neurotransmitter is stored in synaptic vesicles. These vesicles are observed to cluster about the "active zone" of the synapse. The release of transmitter is accomplished by exocytosis: synaptic vesicles fuse with the membrane and dump their contents into the synaptic cleft. The release reaction is linked to calcium entry through special voltage-gated ion channels at the nerve terminal. Katz demonstrated the failure of neuromuscular transmission in the absence of extracellular calcium.

Neurotransmitter is releasd into the synapse in packets, or quanta. Each quantum contains 5,000 to 10,000 molecules of transmitter substance, the contents of a single synaptic vesicle. The postsynaptic membrane shows spontaneous activity in a quiet preparation. Small potentials are recorded at irregular, sporadic intervals. These events average 0.5 mV in amplitude, in contrast to 50 to 60 mV for a typical end plate potential. They are known as miniature end plate potentials

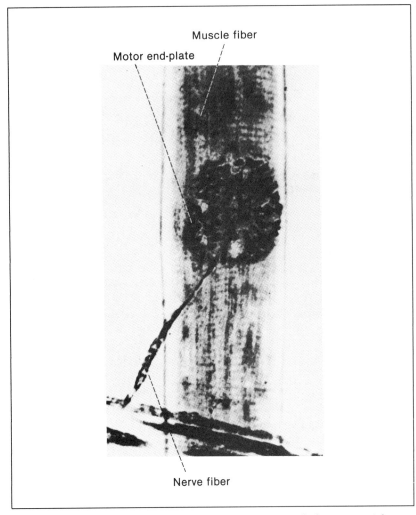

FIGURE 3-2. This photomicrograph shows the motor end plate, a specialized zone along the muscle fiber where the synapse is found. (From R. Snell, *Clinical Neuroanatomy*. Boston: Little, Brown, 1987, p. 129, with permission.)

(mini-EPPs). Mini-EPPs are due to the occasional release of a quantum of neurotransmitter as a single vesicle discharges its contents. This is a random event, merely a source of background noise at the neuromuscular junction. (There is some suggestion that spontaneous release has a tonic effect on the maintenance or tuning of the synapse.)

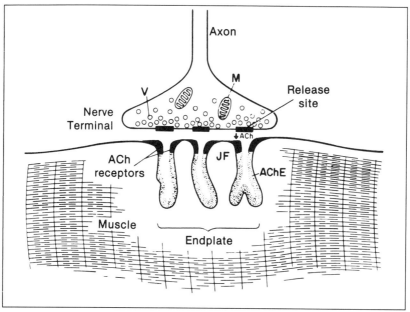

FIGURE 3-3. Schematic diagram of the neuromuscular junction: Vesicles (V) release neurotransmitter molecule at specialized release sites. Receptors for the neurotransmitter acetylcholine (ACh) are densely situated at the top of the junctional folds (JF). Acetylcholinesterase (AChE) rapidly hydrolyzes acetylcholine. M = mitochondria. (From D. Drachman. Myasthenia gravis. *New Eng. J. Med.* 298 : 136, 1978, with permission.)

Acetylcholine

Acetylcholine is made from choline, a ubiquitous nutrient that is a building block of membrane phospholipids. Choline is esterified in nervous tissues by choline acetyltransferase. Otto Loewi in 1921 was the first to appreciate the special role of acetylcholine in nervous transmission. He demonstrated that the effluent of the stimulated vagus nerve could be applied to slow cardiac contraction. Acetylcholine was subsequently identified as the stuff secreted by the vagus, and was shown to be the transmitter substance at the neuromuscular junction by Dale et al. in the 1930s.

When a substance is identified as a neurotransmitter, rigorous criteria must be satisfied: (1) The presence of the putative neurotransmitter must be established in the presynaptic nerve terminal. It is also helpful to identify the machinery for its synthesis and storage. (2) The substance in question must be released with stimulation of the presynaptic neuron. (3) Exogenous administration of the substance must mimic the effect of nerve stimulation, and should do so at the appropriate concentration. This requirement, often called "mimicry," is usually established by microelectrophoresis or micropipetting the substance onto the synapse in an experimental preparation. (4) There should be a predictable effect of the relevant agonist and antagonist drugs on postsynaptic activity. These criteria have been satisfied for acetylcholine at the neuromuscular junction.

The Acetylcholine Receptor

Paul Ehrlich introduced the concept of *receptors* at the turn of the century to explain the potent and selective action of certain drugs and toxins. Specific receptor molecules mediate the effects of neurotransmitter on the postsynaptic neuron. At the neuromuscular junction, the receptor has been identified and localized to the junctional folds in the motor end plate (see Fig. 3-3). A series of folds or pouches in the membrane increase the receptive area of the synapse. The highest concentration of receptor is found at the mouth of the crypt.

Acetylcholine receptor can be found in great abundance in nature in the electrical organ of certain electric fish. This densely innervated tissue is derived embryologically from skeletal muscle. The receptor has been isolated from this source, purified, and characterized chemically through the work of Nachmansohn and Karlin. The acetylcholine receptor is a glycoprotein complex of molecular weight 275,000 embedded in the cell membrane. It is roughly funnel-shaped, with the ion channel at its center (Fig. 3-4). The complex is composed of five subunits (two alpha, one beta, one gamma, and one delta) of molecular weight 40,000 to 64,000. The molecule's tertiary and quaternary structure is now partially understood, especially in the doughnut-shaped area surrounding the ion channel. Two molecules of acetylcholine bind, one each, to a site on the alpha subunit, inducing a conformational change. The binding of acetylcholine opens the ion channel. The chemically gated ion channel in the receptor is distinct from the voltage-gated sodium channel found elsewhere along the membrane. It is somewhat larger in diameter, allowing larger cations (Ca^{2+}, NH_4^+) to pass in addition to Na^+ and K^+. A preponderance of negative charge at the mouth of the channel effectively excludes anions.

Numa and associates in Kyoto have identified the gene segment which encodes the four subunits for the acetylcholine receptor. The gene for electroplax acetylcholine receptor has been sequenced, a remarkable accomplishment (Fig. 3-5). Pure receptor has been produced from its DNA segment in the laboratory. The receptor at the human neuromuscular junction is thought to be substantially identical.

The receptor complex determines the influence of a neurotransmitter on the postsynaptic target cell. Acetylcholine is excitatory at the neuromuscular junction. At a few sites in the mammalian CNS,

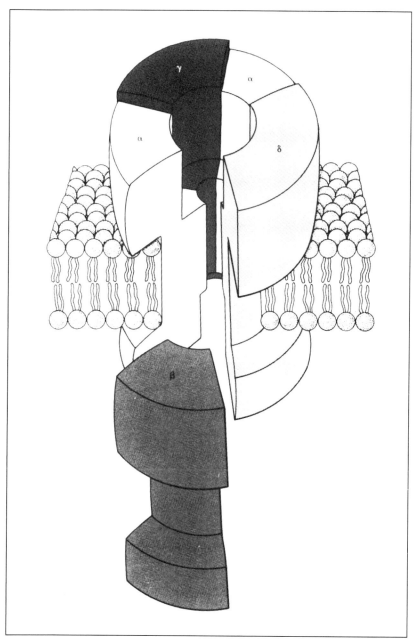

FIGURE 3-4. Three-dimensional model of the nicotinic acetylcholine receptor. Receptor is a funnel-shaped molecule, embedded in the membrane's lipid bilayer. At its core is the ion channel. Receptor complex is composed of five subunits, each of which spans the membrane. (From E.R. Kandel and J.H. Schwartz [eds.], *Principles of Neural Science.* New York: Elsevier, 1985, p. 161, with permission.)

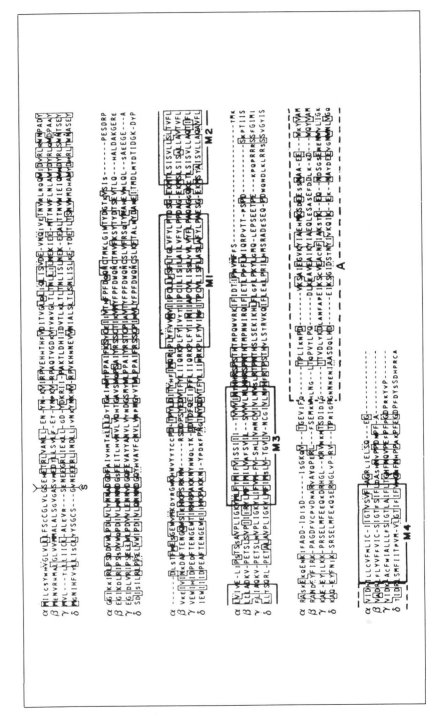

acetylcholine has an inhibitory effect. A different version of the receptor molecule is coupled indirectly to a potassium channel, yielding an inhibitory postsynaptic potential (IPSP). It is not unheard of for the same messenger molecule to have different effects. At the crustacean neuromuscular synapse, GABA is the excitant neurotransmitter. In the mammalian CNS, the same transmitter (GABA) is generally coupled to a chloride ion channel, and is inhibitory. At many sites, the neurotransmitter receptor complex contains no built-in ion channel. The activated receptor effects change indirectly through a second messenger. The β-adrenergic receptor is an example. Norepinephrine attaches to its receptor, and activates a transducer *G protein* in the membrane wall. G protein, in turn, interacts with adenyl cyclase to produce cAMP, an intracellular second messenger. A few of the principal neurotransmitter types are listed in Table 3-1 (see pp. 63–65), along with information about their location and pharmacology.

The interaction of a molecule of acetylcholine with its receptor is a chance event. The amplitude of the electric response (the end plate potential) depends on the number of acetylcholine molecules bound by receptor. There are roughly 10,000 acetylcholine molecules per quantum, and 150 to 200 quanta are released under normal circumstances when the nerve terminal is depolarized. This liberates 2×10^6 neurotransmitter molecules into the synaptic cleft. There are 3 to 4 $\times$ 10^7 receptors waiting at the junctional folds. Only a small number of acetylcholine molecules and receptors interact, the number of "hits" being a matter of chance. Normally 2.5×10^5 ion channels open, producing an end plate potential of 60 mV. This is more than adequate to exceed threshold. The excess of receptor events relative to the minimum necessary to elicit an action potential is known as the *safety margin* for neuromuscular transmission. Any change in the neuromuscular junction, either presynaptic or postsynaptic, that reduces the number of interactions decreases the safety margin and increases the probability of a failure. This is the cardinal principle of neuromuscular transmission.

FIGURE 3-5. Amino acid sequences (deduced from complementary DNA clones) of the alpha, beta, gamma, and delta subunits of the acetylcholine receptor of *Torpedo californica*, as described by Numa et al. (see *Nature* 299 : 793–797, 1982, and 302 : 528–532, 1983). Areas with identical amino acid positions are enclosed by light solid lines. Substantial amino acid homology is evident. The four transmembrane alpha helices are enclosed by heavy lines. (From J.P. Changeux, A. Devillers-Thiery, and P. Chemouille. Acetylcholine receptor: An allosteric protein. *Science* 225 [Sept. 21] : 1338, 1984; © American Association for the Advancement of Science.)

Termination of the Synaptic Effect of Acetylcholine

The effect of acetylcholine at the neuromuscular junction is rapid in onset and brief in duration. The synapse is "on" for only a few milliseconds, the blink of an ion channel. The influence of acetylcholine is limited by diffusion out of the synaptic cleft and by enzymatic hydrolysis. Diffusion of acetylcholine molecules away from the receptor is enhanced by the deep junctional folds. The depth of the folds is sparsely populated with receptors, suggesting that it acts as a sink for synaptically released transmitter. Hydrolysis of acetylcholine by cholinesterase is also important in terminating the synaptic effect. A specific acetylcholinesterase is found in the synapse, while a non-specific or false cholinesterase (butyrylcholinesterase) is found in plasma and non-neural tissues. The true cholinesterase has an anionic and esteratic site to bind acetylcholine. Its structure-activity relationship was described by Nachmansohn and colleagues in the 1960s. It was perhaps the first enzyme to be understood at this level of detail.

MYASTHENIA GRAVIS

This illness was first described in the nineteenth century, though its mechanism was not understood until fairly recently. Patients complain of weakness (asthenia) and fatigue. Fatigue is brought on by exertion and relieved by rest. Symptoms vary over the course of the day. In about 40 percent of cases, initial manifestations are purely ocular. Patients experience drooping of the lids (ptosis) or double vision. Bulbar muscle involvement can lead to nasal speech and difficulty swallowing. Generalized weakness of the limbs develops in about half the cases. Occasionally there is involvement of respiratory muscles and difficulty breathing (gravis).

The problem was localized to the neuromuscular junction through the work of Mary Walker, a resident in neurology, in 1934. Knowledge of the action of acetylcholine at the neuromuscular synapse was then current and widely discussed. She decided to test the response of myasthenic patients to the drug physostigmine, a competitive inhibitor of cholinesterase enzyme. (Cholinesterase inhibitors enhance the synaptic availability of acetylcholine. Physostigmine is used to facilitate neuromuscular transmission, and to help overcome the symptoms of curare poisoning.) This drug produced a miraculous improvement in patients, though the benefits were transient and the myasthenia reappeared when the medication wore off. This simple but elegant human experiment established myasthenia as a disorder of neuromuscular transmission.

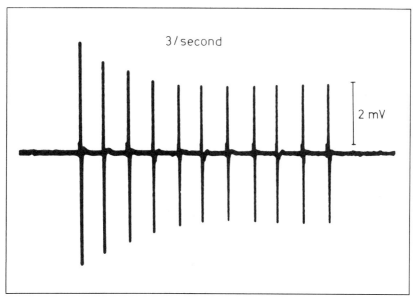

FIGURE 3-6. Decremental response to repetitive nerve stimulation in a patient with myasthenia gravis. Surface electromyogram is recorded from the abductor digiti minimi manus muscle, as the ulnar nerve is stimulated at 3 times per second. Note the characteristic decline in amplitude. (From J.W. Lance and J.G. MacLeod, *A Physiological Approach to Clinical Neurology.* Stoneham, Mass.: Butterworth, 1981, p. 61, with permission.)

Presynaptic or Postsynaptic?

Where is the lesion of the neuromuscular junction in myasthenia? In an attempt to answer this question, investigators looked once again to the physiology. Harvey and co-workers demonstrated a *decremental response* to repetitive nerve stimulation in myasthenic patients. In normals, muscle is able to fire at more than 15 times per second without exhausting the synaptic mechanism. In myasthenia, stimulation at 2 to 5 times per second produces a muscle potential of decreasing amplitude, as more and more junctional synapses fail (Fig. 3-6). This effect may be related to muscle fatigue during sustained use, a prominent complaint in myasthenic patients. Repeated firing does release somewhat less transmitter from the nerve terminal (i.e., fewer packets). In the normal muscle, the inherent safety margin is adequate to prevent a failure. In myasthenic muscle the safety margin of neuromuscular transmission is apparently marginal. Either a presynaptic or a postsynaptic lesion could produce this effect (the probability of an interaction depends equally on the availability of neurotransmitter and receptor).

In 1964 Elmqvist studied intercostal muscle of myasthenic patients using an intracellular recording electrode. He established that the randomly occurring mini-EPPs were smallish in amplitude. At first consideration, this curious result suggests fewer acetylcholine molecules in each terminal vesicle (small quanta). In point of fact, the result merely indicates fewer transmitter-receptor interactions (hits), and fewer open ion channels. This outcome (fewer interactions) could be the product of smaller quanta, as originally suggested by Elmqvist, but a reduced receptor population could have an identical effect.

A definitive localization within the synapse was achieved through the use of a specific marker for the acetylcholine receptor. α-Bungarotoxin is derived from the venom of the Formosan krait, one of a family of poisonous snakes that paralyzes its prey. (A number of biologic toxins appear to act on the neuromuscular junction, a system upon which vertebrate species are universally reliant.) Bungarotoxin binds to the acetylcholine receptor specifically, with high affinity, in an irreversible manner. Radioactive iodine–labeled bungarotoxin can be used to mark acetylcholine receptors in tissue.

Drachman in 1973 applied α-bungarotoxin to muscle biopsy specimens from 10 myasthenic patients. A 70 to 90 percent reduction in receptor number was observed, a dramatic result sufficient in magnitude to account for all the myasthenic phenomena. Morphologic studies subsequently documented a postsynaptic abnormality: a reduction in the junctional folds at the motor end plate. Myasthenia gravis was thus finally identified as a postsynaptic disorder.

Immunopathogenesis of Myasthenia

The next insight into myasthenia came from Patrick and Lindstrom, who were attempting to make antibody to acetylcholine receptor in the laboratory. The receptor is a large glycoprotein complex, an ideal target for antibody production. They used a purified preparation of receptor from the electric eel, and were planning to harvest antibody from rabbits. To their surprise, the rabbits with antibodies became ill; they developed droopy ears and generalized muscular weakness. Patrick and Lindstrom had inadvertently developed an experimental animal model for human myasthenia.

Subsequent studies of human patients with myasthenia demonstrated antibodies to acetylcholine receptor in 87 percent. Patrick and Lindstrom reasoned that the antibodies were the causal factor in the human disease. Yet there was a relatively poor correlation between the patients' antibody titer and their clinical status. Were the antibodies important, or could they be a secondary phenomenon related to receptor injury?

Two observations help to confirm the causal relationship between antireceptor antibody and clinical myasthenia. Pooled serum from myasthenic patients was injected into mice, in order to demonstrate that the illness can be transferred. This study succeeded in producing a myasthenic syndrome in the mice, satisfying the immunologic equivalent of Koch's postulates. The second observation relates to myasthenia in neonates. Children born of myasthenic mothers are often observed to have weakness (neonatal myasthenia). This syndrome persists 30 to 40 days after birth, gradually resolves, and does not recur in later life. Neonatal myasthenia is due to passive transfer of acetylcholine receptor antibodies (IgG class) in utero. When the maternal antibodies are gone from the child's circulation, the illness goes away.

Acetylcholine receptors in skeletal muscle are a dynamic population. Studies with α-bungarotoxin labeling demonstrate a normal receptor turnover of 4 percent per hour; more than half the receptors are replaced in a 24-hour period. The synthesis of receptor is normal in the myasthenic, but the degradation is increased by at least a factor of 2. The antibodies act by marking the receptor for accelerated degradation. As the population of receptors declines, a disorder of neuromuscular transmission results.

Knowledge of the immune cause of myasthenia has extended the range of treatment options. Anticholinesterase medications are often poorly tolerated because of their effects on the autonomic nervous system. They often produce incomplete relief, and a little double vision is as disconcerting as a lot! Chronic excess can block down the neuromuscular junction, and cause a "cholinergic crisis." Systemic steroids are commonly used to treat ocular myasthenia, and may induce a satisfactory remission. Patients with severe myasthenia usually respond to removal of antibody by plasmapheresis.

Cell-mediated immunity also appears to play some role in myasthenia. The disease is associated with a tumor of the thymus gland in 10 percent of cases. Even in the absence of thymoma, the cellular architecture of the thymus is altered. Improvement is commonly observed in patients when the thymus is removed. Thymectomy is sometimes used as a treatment for generalized myasthenia.

OTHER CHOLINERGIC SYSTEMS

We have considered the neuromuscular junction as a model of the cholinergic synapse, but it is not the only cholinergic synapse in the nervous system. Recurrent collaterals from the alpha motor neuron make a synapse within the anterior horn onto the Renshaw cell. The motor neuron uses acetylcholine as a neurotransmitter, and this recurrent synapse is also cholinergic. Acetylcholine is the principal neurotransmitter at autonomic ganglia. In the craniosacral (parasympathetic) division of the autonomic nervous system, acetylcholine is the transmitter for the postganglionic neuron. The effects of the vagus nerve on cardiac muscle and on gastric parietal cells are mediated by acetylcholine.

In the CNS, acetylcholine is the principal neurotransmitter for the brainstem reticular formation and a number of forebrain pathways. The reticular system is discussed in the context of arousal and consciousness (see Chap. 6). Cholinergic nuclei in the septal area and basal forebrain provide a system of projections to the limbic system and cerebral cortex. A map of acetylcholine neurons and their distribution in the nervous system is found in Figure 3-7.

Multiple Receptor Species (Subtypes)

It is sometimes necessary to postulate the existence of multiple classes of receptor for a single neurotransmitter. This phenomenon is well described for dopamine and norepinephrine. Multiple receptors are also described for acetylcholine. The evidence derives from the diverse physiologic and pharmacologic effects observed at different synaptic sites. Acetylcholine is excitatory at the mammalian neuromuscular junction; the receptor contains a cation channel that admits sodium ion when bound. At some sites in the CNS, acetylcholine is associated with presynaptic inhibition. In this case, receptor is coupled with a G protein, which increases membrane permeability to potassium ion. At the neuromuscular junction, the action of acetylcholine is rapid in onset and milliseconds in duration. In the autonomic nervous system, the effect on smooth muscle of the bladder wall and on the salivary gland is measured in seconds. This longer temporal course generally implies an effect mediated by second messenger.

The strongest evidence for multiple cholinergic receptor types comes from the pharmacology: the effects of toxins and drugs. The acetylcholine receptor is divided into two principal types, *nicotinic* and *muscarinic,* based on the response to the plant alkaloids nicotine and muscarine. Dixon in 1907 demonstrated that muscarine mimics the effects of vagal stimulation. Atropine specifically antagonizes the effect of acetylcholine at the muscarinic receptors in the parasympathetic division of the autonomic nervous system. Neither muscarine nor atropine has effects at the neuromuscular junction.

The medicinal effects of nicotine were discovered by the North American Indians, who used tobacco for a variety of medical and ritual purposes. Nicotine was isolated from tobacco as the active ingredient in 1843. Its effects on neuromuscular transmission are rarely seen

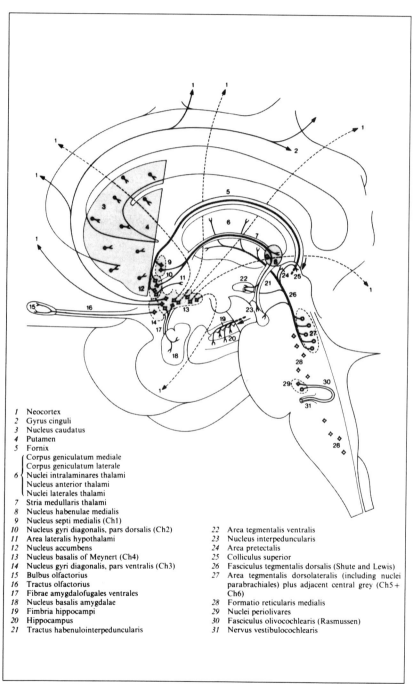

1   Neocortex
2   Gyrus cinguli
3   Nucleus caudatus
4   Putamen
5   Fornix
6   { Corpus geniculatum mediale
      Corpus geniculatum laterale
      Nuclei intralaminares thalami
      Nucleus anterior thalami
      Nuclei laterales thalami
7   Stria medullaris thalami
8   Nucleus habenulae medialis
9   Nucleus septi medialis (Ch1)
10 Nucleus gyri diagonalis, pars dorsalis (Ch2)
11 Area lateralis hypothalami
12 Nucleus accumbens
13 Nucleus basalis of Meynert (Ch4)
14 Nucleus gyri diagonalis, pars ventralis (Ch3)
15 Bulbus olfactorius
16 Tractus olfactorius
17 Fibrae amygdalofugales ventrales
18 Nucleus basalis amygdalae
19 Fimbria hippocampi
20 Hippocampus
21 Tractus habenulointerpeduncularis

22 Area tegmentalis ventralis
23 Nucleus interpeduncularis
24 Area pretectalis
25 Colliculus superior
26 Fasciculus tegmentalis dorsalis (Shute and Lewis)
27 Area tegmentalis dorsolateralis (including nuclei
      parabrachiales) plus adjacent central grey (Ch5 +
      Ch6)
28 Formatio reticularis medialis
29 Nuclei periolivares
30 Fasciculus olivocochlearis (Rasmussen)
31 Nervus vestibulocochlearis

FIGURE 3-7. Cholinergic cell groups and pathways in the CNS. (From R. Nieuwenhuys. *Chemoarchitecture of the Brain.* New York: Springer-Verlag, 1985, p. 8, with permission.)

TABLE 3-1. Neurotransmitter Receptors in the Central Nervous System and Their Receptor Subtypes

Receptor Type	Characteristics
Adrenergic	
α_1	Located postsynaptically in both sympathetic nervous system and brain (where it is found on both neurons and blood vessels). Produces vasoconstriction. Agonist potency: EPI > NE > ISO. Prazosin is a selective antagonist.
α_2	Mostly presynaptic autoreceptor (in sympathetic terminals, locus coeruleus) but also postsynaptic (e.g., in pituitary: mediates growth hormone release.) Agonist potency: NE = EPI > ISO. Clonidine is selective agonist; yohimbine is selective antagonist.
β_1	Localized in heart > lung; found regionally in brain. Stimulates heart. Agonist potency: ISO > EPI = NE. Practolol is selective antagonist.
β_2	Localized in lung > heart; found in brain, glia > neurons. Produces bronchodilation, vasodilation. Agonist potency: ISO > EPI > NE. Salbutamol, terbutaline are selective agonists.
Serotonin (5-HT)	Classification still controversial.
5-HT$_1$	Three subtypes:
5-HT$_{1A}$	Found in gut and dorsal raphe nucleus in various species. Appears to mediate contraction in gut, neuronal inhibition in brain. Spiperone is antagonist; the anxiolytic buspirone is partial agonist.
5-HT$_{1B}$	Found in cortex and sympathetic nervous system. Mediates contraction of smooth muscle and neuronal inhibition.
5HT$_{1C}$	Found in stomach; mediates contraction.
5-HT$_2$	Found in brain, platelets, gut, uterus. Downregulated by antidepressant treatment. Mediates "serotonin syndrome." Methysergide, cyproheptadine, and ketanserine are antagonists.
5-HT$_3$	At least three subtypes exist, all found peripherally. Stimulation causes neuronal depolarization (transmitter release, nociception).
Dopamine	Two types; evidence for others poor.
D$_1$	Located in parathyroid, not pituitary. Present on intrinsic neurons of corpus striatum and in retina. Physiologic role poorly understood.
D$_2$	Located in anterior pituitary (inhibits prolactin release) and on neurons receiving nigrostriatal and mesolimbic dopamine projections. Probably responsible for therapeutic effects of antipsychotics and extrapyramidal effects. Bromocriptine selective agonist. Butyrophenones (e.g., haloperidol) selective antagonists.

Histamine Two types:

H₁ — Found in brain, mast cells. Mediates bronchoconstriction. Antagonists cause drowsiness. Antagonists include classic antihistamines (e.g., diphenhydramine) and some tricyclic antidepressants (doxepin, amitriptyline).

H₂ — In brain, probably located in neocortex, hippocampus. In stomach mediates gastric acid secretion. Cimetidine, ranitidine clinically important antagonists.

Muscarinic–cholinergic — Antagonized by atropine-like drugs, but also by tricyclic antidepressants, many antihistamines, and low-potency neuroleptics, resulting in side effects. Loss of muscarinic-cholinergic transmission in Alzheimer's disease may be partly responsible for cognitive decline. Two types generally recognized pharmacologically, but four types predicted by cloning.

M₁ — Located in sympathetic ganglia, frontal cortex, corpus striatum, hippocampus.

M₂ — Located in brainstem, cerebellum, heart. Recently shown to open a K⁺ channel by a G protein–linked mechanism causing hyperpolarization and therefore bradycardia.

Adenosine — Two types, A₁ and A₂. In brain, adenosine inhibits transmitter release. Adenosine agonists are sedating and anxiolytic. The behavioral-stimulant effects of xanthines such as caffeine are due to blockade of adenosine receptors. Peripherally agonists produce vasodilation.

Opiate — At least three types; naloxone is an antagonist at all types with affinity: μ › δ › κ.

mu (μ) — Localized in periaqueductal gray, thalamus, substantia gelatinosa of spinal cord, and other regions. Mediates analgesia and indifference to pain, miosis, and respiratory depression. Morphine and related opiate alkaloids are exogenous agonists; β-endorphin and the enkephalins are endogenous agonists.

delta (δ) — Highest density in limbic system. Mediates analgesia, hypotension, and miosis. Enkephalins are endogenous agonists. No selective agonists in clinical use because only peptide agonists known.

kappa (κ) — Located in deep cortical layers. Mediates sedating analgesia, miosis. Benzomorphan drugs, e.g., ketamine, pentazocine, selective agonists. Dynorphins are the endogenous agonists.

Sigma (σ) — Formerly considered to be an opiate receptor because it binds the opiate-like drug, SKF 10,047, but unlike opiate receptors it is insensitive to naloxone. Haloperidol, but not all antipsychotics, is an antagonist at this site. The function and endogenous ligand, if any, are unknown.

PCP (phencyclidine) — Although not originally distinguished from the sigma receptor, this receptor is insensitive to both naloxone and haloperidol. It is the site of action of the psychotomimetic compound phencyclidine (PCP). It appears to be a site within the NMDA receptor channel. Blockade of this channel may protect against neuronal death during hypoglycemia, anoxia. Experimental drug MK 801, which acts at this site, now being tested for these indications.

TABLE 3-1 (Continued).

Receptor Type	Characteristics
Excitatory amino acids	The match between ligand (glutamate, aspartate, or some other amino acid) and these receptors not yet clear. Nomenclature is in flux; most commonly used names are based on distinguishing agonists.
N-methyl-D-aspartate (NMDA), or A_1	Not involved in classic fast synaptic transmission. High concentration in hippocampus, cortex. May be important in learning and memory and in pathogenesis of epilepsy and hypoglycemic, anoxic damage. Effects antagonized by PCP, MK801, which block its effector channel.
Quisqualate, or A_2	Glutamate has a higher affinity than aspartate at this receptor. Along with kainate receptors, these mediate classic (fast) excitatory synaptic transmission in brain.
Kainate, or A_3	Endogenous ligand unclear. High concentration in limbic system. Like quisqualate receptor, mediates fast excitatory synaptic transmission.
GABA	Two types:
GABA $_A$	Mediates classic inhibitory transmission in higher brain centers. (Glycine serves this purpose in the brainstem and spinal cord.) Thus receptors found on majority of neurons in forebrain. The receptor acts through an intrinsic chloride channel. The receptor also contains binding sites for benzodiazepines and barbiturates. Binding of these drugs increases the affinity of the receptor for GABA. Muscimol is a selective agonist; bicuculline (proconvulsant) is an antagonist.
GABA$_B$	Works through G proteins, not C1 channel (nonclassic effect). Baclofen is selective agonist.

Key: EPI = epinephrine; NE = norepinephrine; ISO = isoproterenol; 5-HT = 5-hydroxytryptamine; NMDA = N-methyl-*d*-aspartate; GABA = γ-aminobutyric acid. Source: Modified from S.E. Hyman, Neurotransmitter receptors. *Psychosomatics* 29 : 256–257, 1988.

clinically, as it has potent effects on the autonomic ganglia. The quantity of nicotine contained in two or three cigarettes would be a fatal dose, if ingested and fully absorbed. In reality, the autonomic effects of nicotine induce vomiting before a large amount can be absorbed orally. According to the Surgeon General's report, nicotine from cigarette smoke has powerful addictive effects on the CNS, comparable to opiates and cocaine. It is known to induce phenomena of tolerance and withdrawal at the autonomic ganglia. In one study by Schachter et al., smokers switching to a cigarette with a lower nicotine content were observed to increase the frequency and depth of their inhalation, as if to regulate their nicotine dose and blood level.

Curare, a substance discovered by South American Indians, specifically antagonizes the effect of acetylcholine at the nicotinic receptor. It was originally used on poison-tipped darts and spears to cause paralysis, but has found a more civilized application in anesthesia. Nicotine and curare do not cross-react to any appreciable degree with muscarinic receptors. There is some evidence that the nicotinic receptors in the autonomic ganglia differ from those at the neuromuscular junction. α-Bungarotoxin binds poorly and does not block receptors at the autonomic ganglion. The antagonists hexamethonium and decamethonium have differential effects at the two sites.

Both muscarinic and nicotinic cholinergic synapses are found in the CNS, where the muscarinic type predominates. There is bungarotoxin binding in the CNS, but it is weak and its significance is unclear.

PHARMACOLOGY OF THE SYNAPSE AT THE NEUROMUSCULAR JUNCTION

Knowledge of synaptic mechanisms and the influence of drugs on the synapse is important in medicine. Many diseases and biologic toxins produce their effects on the nervous system at the synapse. Myasthenia gravis is a good example. The pharmacology of the neuromuscular junction is also important in anesthesia, where paralyzing agents are routinely administered. The pharmacology gives us a therapeutic lever with which to reduce deficits and improve nervous system function. Drugs that influence synaptic mechanisms provide a basis for therapeutics in neurology and psychiatry. As an example, Alzheimer's disease is a disease of the brain which causes dementia. Pathologic examination shows marked involvement of cholinergic systems in the basal forebrain. Drugs which directly or indirectly augment cholinergic function have been used as the basis for experimental therapy of Alzheimer's disease.

Figure 3-8 is a simplified schematic of the cholinergic synapse. Using this diagram, we will review the sites at which various drugs and toxins have an effect on the neuromuscular junction:

Site 1. The choline acetyltransferase enzyme is particular to nerve terminals that utilize acetylcholine as a synaptic transmitter. It is a biochemical marker for the cholinergic synapse. Styryl pyridine derivatives can block the synthesis of acetylcholine in the laboratory, but there are no practical therapeutic options at this site.

Site 2. The release of acetylcholine is calcium-dependent. The synapse will not function in a calcium-free medium. The agents 3,4-diaminopyridine and guanidine facilitate the release reaction. As noted above, the pharmacology of the mammalian neuromuscular junction is steeped in the folklore of biologic toxins. β-Bungarotoxin and black widow spider venom promote release. These toxins may dump enough acetylcholine into the synapse to cause a depolarizing block. The release reaction is antagonized by botulinum toxin. Botulinum toxin is sometimes used therapeutically to reduce excessive muscle contraction in focal dystonic disorders.

Two clinical disorders of neuromuscular transmission are expressed at this site. *Botulism* is a rare but serious illness caused by the toxin elaborated by the bacterium *Clostridium botulinum*. Both wound and foodborne infections are described. The bacteria grow especially well in home-bottled preserves. Weakness appears first in cranial muscles as dysarthria, diplopia, and dysphagia. Dry mouth suggests involvement of the parasympathetics. Respiratory support may be necessary while the toxin is cleared. Infant botulism is often more subtle, presenting with bulbar weakness and a floppy baby.

The *Eaton-Lambert syndrome* is a presynaptic disorder of neuromuscular transmission observed in patients with small-cell carcinoma of the lung. It is presently unclear what the cancer elaborates to interfere with the function of the nerve terminal. The release of acetylcholine is diminished. Unlike myasthenics, patients with Eaton-Lambert syndrome show an initial incrementing response to repetitive nerve stimulation (Fig. 3-9). The defect in acetylcholine release in Eaton-Lambert syndrome and in botulism is treated with 3,4-diaminopyridine or with guanidine.

Site 3. The nicotinic receptor in the postsynaptic junctional folds is an obvious site for intervention. Nicotine is an agonist in experimental studies of the neuromuscular junction, though the autonomic effects of nicotine predominate clinically. Curare, a pure antagonist, and succinylcholine, a depolarizing blocker, are used in anesthesia. Rabies virus is thought to have its CNS and autonomic effects on the nicotinic

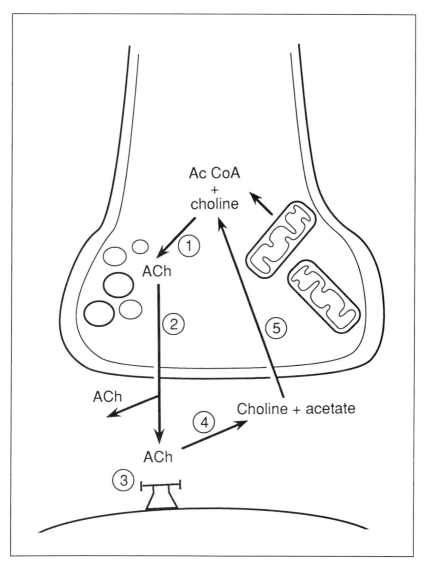

Figure 3-8. Schematic diagram of the cholinergic synapse, illustrating sites of drug action: (1) Acetylcholine synthesis can be blocked by styryl pyridine derivatives. (2) Release is promoted by β-bungarotoxin and black widow spider venom. Release is blocked by botulinum toxin and Mg^{2+}. (3) Postsynaptic receptors are of two types: nicotinic and muscarinic. Nicotinic receptors are blocked by α-bungarotoxin, rabies virus, and curare. Muscarinic receptors are blocked by atropine and quinuclidinyl benzilate (QNB). (4) Acetylcholinesterase is inhibited reversibly by physostigmine, pyridostigmine, and edriphonium, irreversibly by diisopropyl fluorophosphate (DFP). (5) Competitive blockers of choline uptake include hemicholinium-3. (Adapted from J.R. Cooper and F.E. Bloom. *Biochemical Basis of Neuropharmacology* [5th ed.]. New York: Oxford University Press, 1986. P. 197.)

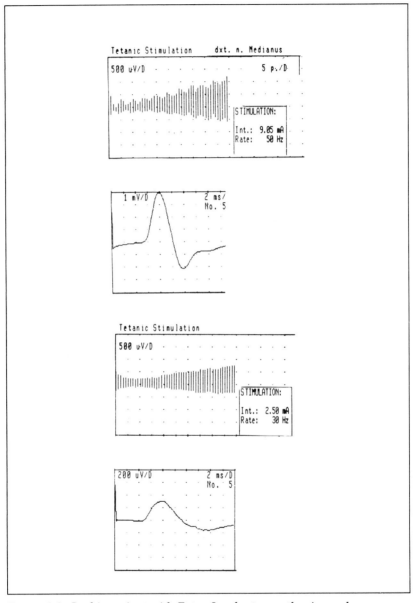

FIGURE 3-9. In this patient with Eaton-Lambert myasthenic syndrome, thenar hand muscles are recorded during high-frequency stimulation of the median nerve. At a stimulation rate of 30 times per second, there is an *incremental* response as the presynaptic defect is overcome. The change is even more apparent at a stimulation rate of 50 times per second. Over the course of the study, the amplitude of the motor potential increases from 0.5 mV (*left*) to almost 4 mV (*right*). (Courtesy of Dr. Jeremy Shefner, Brigham and Women's Hospital, Boston.)

receptor. Rabies infection stimulates a great deal of salivation. Behavioral effects of limbic system infection with rabies promote the transmission of the virus.

Site 4. Acetylcholinesterase is responsible for the hydrolysis of acetylcholine, and contributes to the termination of the synaptic effect. Cholinesterase inhibitors such as physostigmine are used to antagonize curare and reverse neuromuscular paralysis. Response to edriphonium, a short-acting cholinesterase inhibitor, is used as a diagnostic test for myasthenia. Before edriphonium is administered, the patient is usually pretreated with atropine to block the autonomic effects.

Diisopropyl fluorophosphate (DFP) is one of several organophosphorus agents commonly found in insecticides. These chemicals irreversibly antagonize cholinesterase, and have a more profound autonomic and neuromuscular effect. Compounds have been devised for chemical warfare (nerve gas) which act on cholinesterase.

Site 5. The production of acetylcholine is dependent on the constant bioavailability of choline. Presynaptic nerve terminals have a site for high-affinity choline uptake. Oral choline or lecithin (phosphatidylcholine) is used to promote the synthesis and release of acetylcholine. These treatments have little effect on neuromuscular transmission, but may influence cholinergic systems in the CNS. Hemicholinium-3 and triethylcholine are antagonists of choline uptake, but these drugs are not used clinically.

The pharmacology of the synapse provides us with a degree of control over events at the neuromuscular junction. A similar knowledge of the dopamine synapse has been important in neurology for the treatment of Parkinson's disease. Many of the drugs presently used in psychiatric practice have effects on dopamine, norepinephrine, or serotonin. Further therapeutic advances await better characterization of synaptic mechanisms for other neurotransmitters.

BIBLIOGRAPHY

Drachman, D.B. Myasthenia gravis. *N. Engl. J. Med.* 298:136–142, 186–193, 1978.

Goodman, L., and Gilman, A. *The Pharmacological Basis of Therapeutics* (7th ed.). New York: Macmillan, 1985. Chaps. 4, 6, 9.

Katz, B. *Nerve, Muscle, and Synapse.* New York: McGraw-Hill, 1966.

McCarthy, M.P., et. al. The molecular biology of the acetylcholine receptor. *Annu. Rev. Neurosci.* 9:383–413, 1986.

PART **II**

Sensory-Motor Integration

CHAPTER 4

Pain and Somatic Sensation

We experience our world through the various modalities of sensation. While some senses (vision, hearing, balance, taste, and smell) are confined to highly specialized sense organs, general afferents are widely distributed over the body wall and viscera. They help us to feel pain, to discriminate, and to localize. The nervous system maintains a separate anatomy for two principal categories of general somatic sensation. The posterior column pathway conveys information about tactile discrimination and joint position sense. The anterolateral spinal system concerns itself with pain and temperature. Separate pathways allow for functional specializations, which will be apparent when the two systems are considered in more detail.

PERIPHERAL RECEPTORS AND SEGMENTAL ANATOMY

A network of free nerve endings in skin and soft tissue acts as peripheral receptors for the pain pathway. Free nerve endings can be excited directly by strong pressure or by tissue injury. Chemicals in the extracellular fluid (ECF) can also initiate depolarization of unencapsulated nerve endings. Bradykinin, histamine, acetylcholine, and substance P excite free nerve endings; some of these substances are released into the ECF with tissue injury. High extracellular potassium can depolarize the membrane; ionic potassium is often released after cellular injury.

Special encapsulated receptors exist for hot and cold (Krause's corpuscles), touch (Meissner's corpuscles), pressure and vibration (pacinian corpuscles). They act as transducers, changing the various thermal and mechanical stimuli into electrical signals. Receptors produce the *sensory generator potential*, a depolarization of the afferent nerve ending which reflects stimulus intensity. A train of action potentials in the primary afferent is transmitted proximally. The discharge rate in afferent fibers is highly correlated with the intensity of

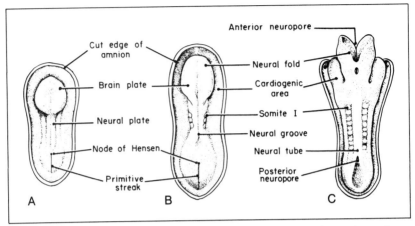

FIGURE 4-1. By the third week of development, axial mesoderm along the neural plate congeals into blocks, or somites. A, B, C = First, second, third weeks of development respectively. (From M.B. Carpenter and J. Sutin, *Human Neuroanatomy,* [8th ed.]. P. 63. © 1985, the Williams & Wilkins Co., Baltimore.)

stimulation. Some receptors, such as the pacinian corpuscles, show rapid adaptation over time.

Segmental Peripheral Anatomy

All first-order sensory afferents have their cell body in the dorsal root ganglion. The segmental peripheral anatomy of sensory systems is a bit peculiar, and derives from the embryology of the neural tube. The axial mesodermal tissue of the embryo congeals into blocks or somites in the third week of development, providing the primitive embryo with some resemblance to a segmented worm (Fig. 4-1). At each segment, the neural crest cells form an intermediate mass, between the neural tube and surface ectoderm. These cell clusters coalesce as the dorsal root ganglia and their processes invade the developing spinal cord. A segmental map of afferent nerves can be projected onto the body wall, where the nerve impulses originate. The map of segmental representation of afferents becomes more complex with the development of the limb buds (Fig. 4-2). A dermatome is that cutaneous area supplied by a single dorsal root and its ganglion.

Sherrington explored the cutaneous map in the monkey and noted an overlap of at least 50 percent with adjacent dermatomes. Section of three contiguous roots was required to produce a distinct band of cutaneous anesthesia. Head studied the dermatomes of man by map-

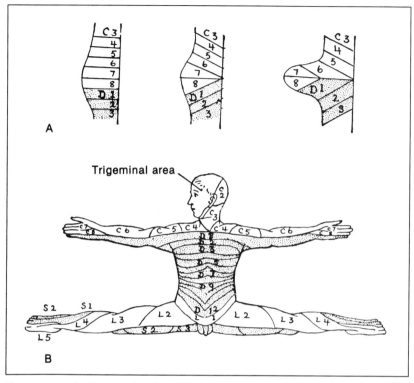

FIGURE 4-2. A. During development of the limbs, segmental representation follows the limb buds in their migration. B. This pattern is reflected in the pattern of the dermatome map along the extremities. (From M.B. Carpenter and J. Sutin, *Human Neuroanatomy* [8th ed.]. © 1985, the Williams & Wilkins Co., Baltimore.)

ping the vesicular eruption of herpes zoster, an infection of the dorsal root ganglion. Dermatome maps obtained by different methods are not entirely congruent. In particular, the dermatomes for pain and temperature are the most narrow. Consequently, examining for altered cutaneous pain perception is the most sensitive method for appreciation of a neurologic deficit involving a single segment.

The dermatome map is valuable as a tool in localization and clinical diagnosis, especially in disorders of the peripheral nervous system (Fig. 4-3). Major landmarks of the sensory map should be remembered. The posterior occiput lies within the top spinal dermatome, C2. C6 encompasses the thumb and index finger; T4 is at the nipple line; T10, the umbilicus; L1, the inguinal ligament; L4, the knee; S1, the sole of the foot; and S3–5, the perianal region. An odd discontinuity of the map on the anterior trunk results from the growth of the upper

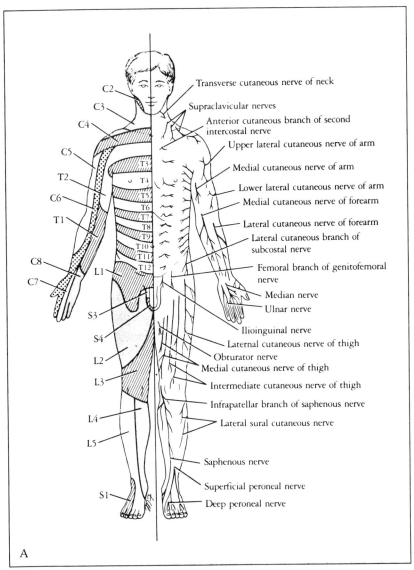

Transverse cutaneous nerve of neck

Supraclavicular nerves

Anterior cutaneous branch of second intercostal nerve

Upper lateral cutaneous nerve of arm

Medial cutaneous nerve of arm

Lower lateral cutaneous nerve of arm

Medial cutaneous nerve of forearm

Lateral cutaneous nerve of forearm

Lateral cutaneous branch of subcostal nerve

Femoral branch of genitofemoral nerve

Median nerve

Ulnar nerve

Ilioinguinal nerve

Laternal cutaneous nerve of thigh

Obturator nerve

Medial cutaneous nerve of thigh

Intermediate cutaneous nerve of thigh

Infrapatellar branch of saphenous nerve

Lateral sural cutaneous nerve

Saphenous nerve

Superficial peroneal nerve

Deep peroneal nerve

A

FIGURE 4-3. The dermatome map of sensory innervation is a valuable tool in diagnosis. (From R. Snell, *Clinical Neuroanatomy for Medical Students.* Boston: Little, Brown, 1987, pp. 150, 151, with permission.)

limb bud. C4 directly opposes T2 on the chest wall. Patterns of sensory loss in the limbs can be seen to conform to the territory of distribution of dermatomes, if the deficit is due to disease of the nerve root or spinal segment.

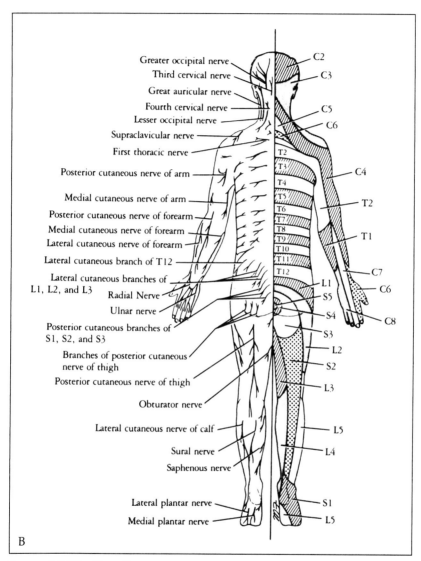

Greater occipital nerve
Third cervical nerve
Great auricular nerve
Fourth cervical nerve
Lesser occipital nerve
Supraclavicular nerve
First thoracic nerve
Posterior cutaneous nerve of arm
Medial cutaneous nerve of arm
Posterior cutaneous nerve of forearm
Medial cutaneous nerve of forearm
Lateral cutaneous nerve of forearm
Lateral cutaneous branch of T12
Lateral cutaneous branches of
L1, L2, and L3
Radial Nerve
Ulnar nerve
Posterior cutaneous branches of
S1, S2, and S3
Branches of posterior cutaneous
nerve of thigh
Posterior cutaneous nerve of thigh
Obturator nerve
Lateral cutaneous nerve of calf
Sural nerve
Saphenous nerve
Lateral plantar nerve
Medial plantar nerve

C2
C3
C5
C6
T2
T3
T4
T5
T6
T7
T8
T9
T10
T11
T12
C4
T2
T1
L1
S5
S4
S3
L2
S2
L3
C7
C6
C8
L5
L4
S1
L5

B

FIGURE 4-3 (Continued).

PAIN

Pain is a signal of enormous biologic importance. Rare individuals born with congenital indifference to pain suffer frequent accidental injury and have difficulty adjusting to their environment. Pain (chest pain, abdominal pain) is an important symptom in general medicine.

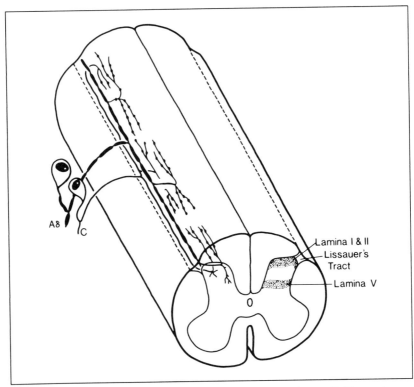

FIGURE 4-4. Note the extensive terminal field of a single small-fiber primary afferent. Fibers bifurcate as they enter the spinal grey, and ascend or descend a few levels in Lissauer's tract. Unmyelinated C fibers terminate primarily in lamina II, while A-delta fibers terminate in laminae I and V. Primary afferents are varicose and longitudinally oriented, contacting hundreds of spinal neurons. (From H.L. Fields, *Pain.* New York: McGraw-Hill, 1987, p. 45, with permission.)

A further measure of the biologic and social import of pain is evident in the more than 300 commercially available over-the-counter analgesics, and the large and lucrative trade in illicit narcotics. In the United States 2 million workers are incapacitated by pain, and compensation payments exceed $2.5 million per year. At the same time, pain is an intensely personal and subjective experience which is difficult to quantitate and study.

The Pain Transmission Pathway

An anatomic system is designed for the central transmission of pain information. It is known as the spinothalamic tract (the anterolateral pathway). It is often thought of as a conduit for sensory messages from pain-specific receptors in the periphery. In reality, however, it is a more complex system with intelligent processing at the brainstem and spinal level. Peripheral inputs converge on the dorsal gray as a richly textured pattern, woven from the fabric of pain and general somatic afferents.

Two classes of afferent nerve fibers convey pain information. Small, poorly myelinated nerve fibers (A-delta class) carry afferent sensory information at 5 to 30 m/sec. Unmyelinated C fibers, under 2 μm in diameter, conduct at only 0.5 to 2.0 m/sec. They are principally concerned with pain and autonomic information. The cell body for all primary sensory afferents lies in the dorsal root ganglion, and the proximal axon segment enters the spinal cord to synapse. Degeneration studies reveal that many afferents ascend or descend a segment or two in the tract of Lissauer prior to synapse (Fig. 4-4).

The dorsal horn is the site of first synapse of primary pain afferents. Substance P is thought to be the neurotransmitter for the C fibers. The synaptic organization of sensory afferents in the dorsal horn is complex; many make contact with local interneurons. The principal projection neurons for the pathway are in laminae I and V of the spinal cord. The marginal cells of lamina I are relatively specific for pain and thermal stimuli. Lamina V cells are wide dynamic-range mechanoreceptors, which also process C fiber input. Their activity reflects a convergence of different afferents (Fig. 4-5).

The neurons in laminae I and V of the dorsal horn send their axons *across the spinal cord* in the anterior white commissure. These fibers collect to ascend in the anterolateral spinal tract (Fig. 4-6). A minority, a phylogenetically older subset of the pathway, remain uncrossed and ascend in the anterior funiculus. Consequently, section of the anterolateral tract does not eliminate all pain-bearing messages from the contralateral side below.

Duality of the Anterolateral System

The term *spinothalamic tract* evokes the image of a tightly organized, coherent ascending projection to the thalamus. In reality, less than half of the spinothalamic afferents reach the thalamus. A majority of afferents in the anterolateral bundle leak out along the way and synapse in the brainstem reticular formation. The reticular formation is responsible for alerting us to the threat of noxious stimuli. In a sense, the anterolateral tract contains two distinct pathways: the proper spinothalamic tract, and a phylogenetically older division, the *spinoreticulothalamic* tract. The older pathway is not strictly somatotopic, and seems to convey diffuse information.

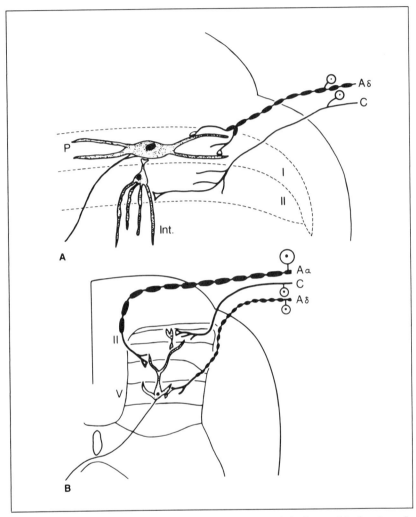

FIGURE 4-5. Dorsal horn projection neurons are mainly located in laminae I and V of the spinal cord. Marginal cells of lamina I are relatively pain-specific. They receive direct input from myelinated A-delta fibers, and indirect input from C fibers, via interneurons in lamina II. Lamina V cells have a convergence of inputs, and display a wide dynamic range. (From H.L. Fields, *Pain.* New York: McGraw-Hill, 1987, p. 55, with permission.)

The fibers of the *neospinothalamic* tract proceed rostrally to synapse in the thalamus. The ventral posterolateral (VPL) and ventral postero-medial (VPM) nuclear groups mediate recognition of pain from the contralateral body and face, respectively. Most of the axons projecting to VPL and VPM originate in cells in laminae I and V with small, crisply focused receptive fields. Messages sent through the reticular

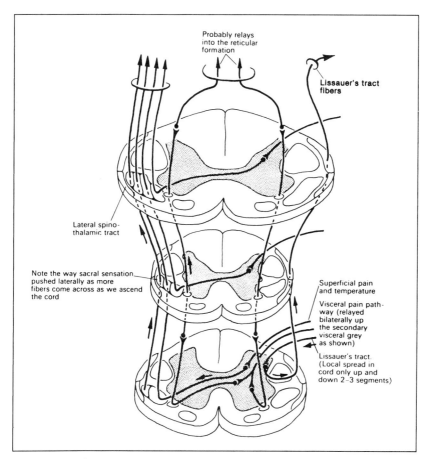

Probably relays into the reticular formation

Lissauer's tract fibers

Lateral spino-thalamic tract

Note the way sacral sensation pushed laterally as more fibers come across as we ascend the cord

Superficial pain and temperature

Visceral pain pathway (relayed bilaterally up the secondary visceral grey as shown)

Lissauer's tract. (Local spread in cord only up and down 2–3 segments)

FIGURE 4-6. The pain transmission pathway: Afferent fibers enter the spinal cord via the dorsal root, and may ascend or descend a few segments in Lissauer's tract. After synapse in the dorsal horn, the pathway crosses to ascend in the anterolateral spinothalamic tract. A small number of fibers remain uncrossed (From J. Patten, *Neurological Differential Diagnosis.* Heidelberg, West Germany: Springer-Verlag, 1978, p. 139, with permission.)

formation terminate in the adjacent intralaminar complex and medial thalamus. Many of these projections originate in the deeper laminae of the spinal cord, in cells with large and complex receptive fields.

Physiologists often speak of two kinds of pain: fast pain and slow pain. Appreciation of pinprick is rapid ("ouch!"), quick to decay, and fairly localizable. A wave of slow, persistent, noxious sensation often follows, which is considerably more diffuse. This is the pain that keeps people awake at night. Slow pain may be said to reside in the C fibers, the spinoreticular pathway, the intralaminar and medial thalamic nuclei.

The VPL and VPM, often called the *ventrobasal complex,* send projections to the SI and SII sensory cortex. Yet, in some sense, pain happens as a mental entity at the level of the thalamus. Cortical ablations do not eliminate pain, a sensory experience which is deeply rooted in conscious awareness. Lesions of VPL compromise pinprick localization, but a deep nagging chronic pain may persist. Lesions of the intralaminar thalamic nuclei may relieve some of the chronic noxiousness of pain, but not cutaneous sensitivity to pinprick. (Oddly, electrical stimulation of the thalamus does not elicit pain. Low-frequency stimulation of the intralaminar thalamic nuclei is reported as analgesic and rather relaxing. This curious observation suggests that the temporospatial pattern of afferents is important in the thalamic appreciation of pain.)

Puzzling Pain Phenomena

The anterolateral system, a model for the pain transmission pathway, formed the basis in the early twentieth century for understanding pain symptoms. The approach to pain was predicated on a knowledge of the segmental peripheral anatomy, and the distribution of the spinothalamic tract. Information derived from the anatomy is accurate and correct, but also incomplete in that it tells only a part of the story. Many common clinical phenomena remain mysterious or poorly understood when analyzed as the production of the anterolateral system.

Pause for a moment to consider the paradox of a painful peripheral neuropathy or nerve injury. Some generalized disorders of peripheral nerve, diabetic neuropathy in particular, can result in a state of chronic pain. Pain is distal, burning in nature, and is particularly bad at night, when other afferent messages are at a low ebb. It is difficult to understand, in terms of the above model, how a pruning of the peripheral pain transmission pathway (loss of axons and Schwann cells) can result in a painful condition. In fact, pain frequently results from damage to somatosensory pathways, anywhere from the peripheral nerve to the thalamus.

The hardest phenomenon for this model to explain is the central modification of pain (descending control). Stress analgesia is described among soldiers in wartime, in whom large tissue injuries are endured without pain for brief periods in the heat of battle. Only later does the patient experience overwhelming pain, even shock commensurate with the injury. A competitor recently finished the Boston marathon, running the last miles on a stress fracture of the femur. This is an extraordinary accomplishment in pain control. Hypnotic analgesia is another example of descending control. In no sense can the brain be considered to be a slave to peripheral impulses; it obviously exerts a unique degree of control over the use of its pain pathways.

The Gate Theory of Pain

Introduced in 1965 by Melzak and Wall, the gate theory was a step forward in understanding pain control. Like many a "patch" used to shore up an existing theory in the face of newer data, it is not strictly correct. It is, however, a helpful advance toward understanding the segmental modification of pain.

Melzak and Wall discussed the pain pathway in terms of a gate-keeper and its influence on the projection neuron *(pain transmission neuron)* in the deeper laminae of the substantia gelatinosa. According to their hypothesis, transmission along the pathway reflects the inter-action between unmyelinated C fibers and myelinated large fiber affer-ents. Either input can directly stimulate the pain transmission cell. In addition, they proposed an inhibitory interneuron (gatekeeper) in lamina II of the substantia gelatinosa, with inhibitory synapse onto the pain transmission cell (Fig. 4-7). In their schema, large fiber affer-ents promote, and unmyelinated axons suppress, this inhibition.

The point of this model is that a barrage of large fiber afferents (from A-alpha and A-beta touch fibers) can act through the interneuron to quiet the activity of the pain pathway. This device is useful to prevent incidental activation of the pain pathway during forceful touching. The predicted wiring diagram for the dorsal horn has not been confirmed by subsequent physiologic studies of the spinal cord in animals. Inhi-bition is important in afferent processing, but the predominant mech-anism appears to be presynaptic inhibition onto C fibers. Yet the detail of the theory is perhaps unimportant. A greater lesson is derived from Melzak and Wall's analysis. The spinothalamic tract is no dedicated slave to peripheral pain afferents. An intelligent network exists within the dorsal horn which monitors peripheral afferents, and decides when to signal the more rostral central nervous system (CNS). The painful message does not reside in pain-specific receptors or nerve fibers, but in the pattern of activation of the dorsal horn.

A productive application of the gate theory has been the develop-ment of the transcutaneous electric nerve stimulator (TENS). This device is applied to the skin over the peripheral nervous system, preferably proximal to the source of pain. The gentle, non-noxious electrical stimulation of large-fiber afferents reduces the amount of pain experienced. These devices afford a considerable measure of re-lief of some patients.

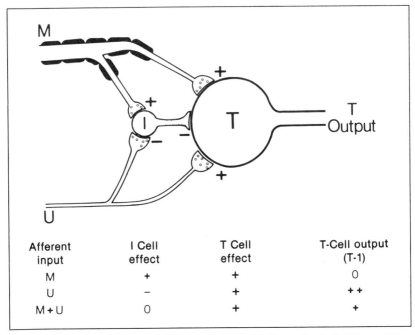

Afferent input	I Cell effect	T Cell effect	T-Cell output (T-1)
M	+	+	0
U	−	+	+ +
M + U	0	+	+

FIGURE 4-7. The gate control theory of pain. This hypothesis focuses upon interactions in the dorsal horn of the spinal cord. The transmission cell (T) controls access to the anterolateral tract. Myelinated large fibers (M) and unmyelinated C fibers (U) both excite the pain transmission cell. An interneuron (I) modulates the activity of the T cell. Large-fiber input tends to promote inhibition of activity in the pain pathway. The table shows how perceived pain (T cell output) is the result of a balance of inputs from myelinated and unmyelinated primary afferents. (From H.L. Fields, *Pain*. New York: McGraw-Hill, 1987, p. 139, with permission.)

The Opiate Receptor

The major advance in our understanding of pain control occurred as recently as 1975, from the study of mechanisms of narcotic analgesia in the laboratory. Derivatives of the opium poppy such as morphine have been available for the relief of pain since the mid-nineteenth century. Opiates, both natural and synthetic, have long been recognized for their analgesic potency. These drugs produce tolerance (a shift in the dose-response curve with chronic use), and withdrawal symptoms occur on their discontinuation.

Several aspects of the pharmacology of the narcotic drugs suggested to Snyder and Pert the possibility of a receptor-mediated effect:

(1) Morphine, heroin, and some of the newer synthetic narcotics are exceedingly potent drugs. These drugs can elicit a biologic response when present in nanomolar concentrations. (2) The molecular specificity of the morphine effect is impressive. The opposite stereoisomer is inactive. (3) There exist highly potent and specific narcotic antagonist drugs. Naloxone differs only slightly from morphine in molecular structure. Yet administration of naloxone can antagonize the effect of morphine specifically on a molecule-for-molecule basis. A small amount of naloxone can precipitate withdrawal in an addict. Following their intuition, Snyder and Pert were able to demonstrate a receptor for morphine in tissues from the vertebrate CNS: a native protein with a high-affinity, specific binding, which mediates the biologic effect of the opiates.

Having discovered the opiate receptor, the next logical step was to question why it was there. Surely the opiate receptor was not placed in nervous tissues to allow the injection of potent synthetic narcotic drugs. Hughes and Kosterlitz pursued their hunch that an endogenous substance was present to interact with the receptor. Within a short period, they discovered two naturally occurring peptides which enjoyed this property. These were dubbed *enkephalin*, from the Greek for "in the head." There are now at least five peptides known to be present in the CNS capable of acting as agonists at the opiate receptor. The principal opiate peptides are met-enkephalin and leu-enkephalin, pentapeptide fragments of naturally occurring α-, β-, and γ-endorphin (Fig. 4-8). β-Endorphin is 50 to 100 times more potent that morphine on a molar basis. These endogenous opiates are all thought to be formed by cleavage from a larger prohormone, β-lipotropin. β-Lipotropin, 91 amino acids in length, is itself inert, though it contains α-, β-, γ-endorphin, and met-enkephalin within it. A network of neurons staining positive for enkephalin by immu-nohistochemistry appears to utilize these compounds as a synaptic transmitter.

The Descending Pain Modification Pathway

At this juncture, a second limb of the pain pathway can be sketched in: the descending pain modification pathway. Opiate receptors are found in the substantia gelatinosa, dorsal raphe nucleus, and the locus ceruleus. Enkephalin-containing neurons can be found in the periaqueductal gray of the midbrain and in the dorsal horn of the spinal cord. The descending pathway can be assembled from these constituent parts. The pathway appears to originate in the periaqueductal gray nucleus of the midbrain, though more rostral control from the

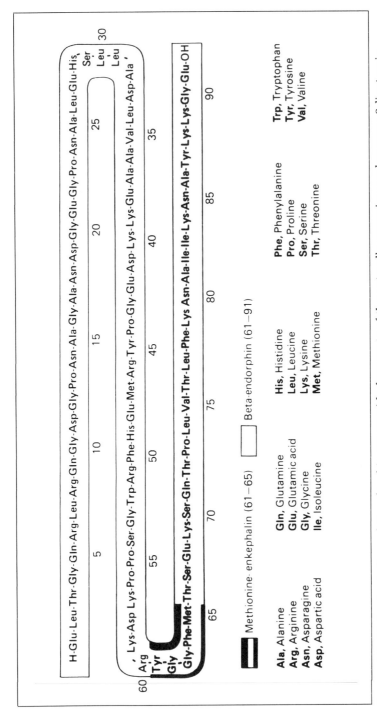

FIGURE 4-8. Met-enkephalin and β-endorphin are peptide fragments of the naturally occurring prohormone β-lipotropin. Met-enkephalin, a pentapeptide, can be seen to reside at positions 61–65. (From E.R. Kandel and J.H. Schwartz [eds.], *Principles of Neural Science* [2nd ed.]. New York: Elsevier, 1985, p. 208, with permission.)

forebrain remains an unconfirmed possibility. The periaqueductal gray contains enkephalin neurons which synapse in the dorsal raphe, a reticular nucleus which projects widely to the neuraxis (Fig. 4-9). Raphe neurons which use serotonin as a principal neurotransmitter descend in the dorsolateral funiculus of the spinal cord, adjacent to the corticospinal and dorsal spinocerebellar tracts. The serotonin cells terminate in the dorsal horn on enkephalin local neurons. Enkephalin neurons synapse on the primary pain afferents as they enter the substantia gelatinosa, causing presynaptic inhibition of pain afferents. The periaqueductal gray can thus modulate afferent pain messages, utilizing a highly specific descending pathway.

How does the network function in pain control? A relevant discovery is the analgesic effect of direct electrical stimulation on the raphe and periaqueductal gray. In animals and in man, stimulation of these brainstem centers produces a high-quality analgesia without sedation. This analgesia has been studied in animals by recording from the dorsal spinal cord during stimulation of the periaqueductal gray. A lamina-specific inhibition is reported, which depresses the activity of pain pathway neurons of laminae I and V *without* changing the activity in adjacent laminae. Narcotics have a similar effect on the spinal cord, though in high doses they have a sedative effect. Midbrain stimulation appears to utilize the descending pathway to elicit a state much like narcotic analgesia.

One can produce a lesion in this pathway by surgical section of the dorsolateral spinal tracts. This lesion blocks stimulation analgesia in segments of the cord ipsilateral to and below the level of the lesion. In animal studies, pharmacologic treatment with serotonin antagonists have the same effect. Naloxone, which antagonizes the effect of narcotics on the segmental appreciation of pain, also blocks stimulation-evoked analgesia. It thus appears that stimulation analgesia and narcotic analgesia are mechanistically similar and utilize the same anatomy.

Placebo Analgesia

In 1979, Fields published a simple and revealing study on the mechanism of the placebo effect. The occasional usefulness of placebos is well known among practicing physicians. Placebos can evoke powerful analgesia, though their clinical use without prior patient consent is an ethically problematic practice. Fields studied pain in dental patients; dental procedures are a consistent source of moderately severe pain. In a group of patients consenting to be studied, 60 percent responded to the placebo as an analgesic following dental work.

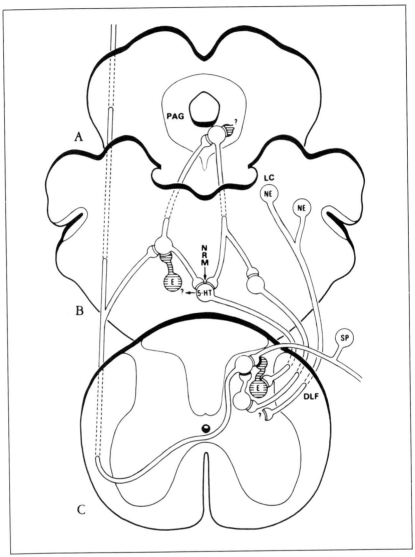

FIGURE 4-9. The descending pain control pathway: Enkephalin-containing neurons are hatched. Endogenous opiate effects are observed at the midbrain (A), lower brainstem (B), and spinal cord (C). They influence function in the periaqueductal gray (PAG) of the midbrain, nucleus raphe magnus (NRM) in the medulla, and substantia gelatinosa of the spinal cord, site of synapse of primary pain afferents (SP). Serotonin projections from the rapha, via the dorsolateral funiculus (DLF), terminate among pain transmission cells. Indirectly, they provide an inhibitory influence on primary pain afferents. Norepinephrine pathways (NE) from the locus ceruleus (LC) also contribute. (From A. Basbaum and H. Fields, Endogenous pain control mechanisms. *Ann. Neurol.* 4 : 455, 1978, with permission.)

These placebo responders received a second drug by intravenous (IV) infusion, either naloxone or saline control. The analgesic effect in the placebo responders was universally antagonized by IV naloxone, but not by saline injection. This elegant study demonstrates that the placebo effect is a very reproducible biologic phenomenon, one which quite likely elicits the endogenous release of opioid peptides. Placebo responders somehow activate the circuits in their periaqueductal gray to effect the release of enkephalin. The 40 percent nonresponders to placebo evidentially cannot access this internal resource.

Strategies for Pain Management

The first step in the successful management of the pain patient is to separate acute from chronic pain. The chronic pain patient, whose pain duration exceeds a year, may be very difficult for complex psychosocial reasons. Pain has become a part of the patient's life to the degree that it may be difficult to separate the patient from his pain. Disability compensation issues are sometimes involved. Short-term pain, such as postoperative pain or pain from trauma, is usually managed satisfactorily with narcotic analgesics. A more difficult problem is the patient with persistent pain from cancer, a problem which has led to a number of strategies. The pain can be treated locally (at its source), through interference with the pain transmission pathway, or by utilizing the descending pain modification pathway.

A half century of neurosurgical literature concerns efforts to relieve pain by producing lesions in the pain transmission pathway. The results of these often mutilating procedures are commonly disappointing. Nerve block can sometimes be used effectively to give relief if the pain is well localized in the distal territory of a single nerve; this result can be made permanent by section of the nerve or injection of a locally toxic agent (alcohol or phenol). Dorsal root section (rhizotomy) is often disappointing, in that analgesia distal to the lesion may be partial and impermanent. Second-order neurons in the dorsal horn develop a pattern of spontaneous, irregular firing, and elements of denervation supersensitivity. Section of the anterolateral spinal tract is also frequently ineffective. Even thalamic surgery is attended by mixed results; a more refractory and diffuse pain may recur late after ablation of the ventrobasal complex. Prefrontal leukotomy and cingulotomy have been occasionally pursued in patients plagued by intolerable pain; but this is personality-altering surgery and as such is generally not done.

Drugs to facilitate the endogenous pain control system have proved a more fruitful strategy for most patients. The effect of moderate non-narcotic analgesics or even narcotic drugs can be enhanced by the simultaneous use of the tricyclic drugs. Amitriptyline increases the synaptic availability of serotonin in the dorsal horn, and thus facilitates the physiologic effect of the descending system. The manipulation of these pathways by drugs that influence synaptic function is a relatively new and promising clinical science.

THE DORSAL COLUMN PATHWAY

Discrete systems exist for the handling of two principal classes of general somatic sensation. Pain and temperature afferents travel the anterolateral system, while joint position and vibration sense are represented in the dorsal column pathway. Information on the status of muscle spindles is relayed to the cerebellum via the dorsal and ventral spinocerebellar tracts. It is unknown whether these tracts produce a conscious sense experience. Cortical modalities are described for various interpreted sense experiences. Examples include stereognosis, the ability to discriminate objects by touch, and graphesthesia, the capacity to understand characters written onto the skin. The diagram below characterizes the structure of somatic sensation as we represent it.

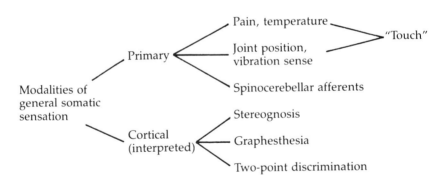

Of course there is something artificial in this analysis. The response to a 128-cps vibration fork is a phenomenon of neurologic examination, and not a physiologic experience. Perhaps vibration receptors helped our ancestors sense the approach of a predator on the jungle floor. Perception of touch, on the other hand, is an important class of sensation. Yet touch is not easily classified as a modality by its physiologic handling. Some crude sense of touch persists after damage to either pathway, while accurate touch localization requires the preservation of the dorsal columns.

There is a philosophical perspective inherent in any theory of somatic sensation. Sensory experience is complex, and understood only as a function of our method of examination and study. Perception is highly subjective, and the reporting of response varies vastly among normal subjects. Data on sensory examination are the least reliable as evidence in neurologic diagnosis. Clinical scientists have tried to define the optimal set of stimuli for complete characterization of somatic sensory systems. The overlap of sensory modalities, particularly the senses with shared cortical representation, is such that any set of examination tools will elicit redundant and perhaps incomplete information. In sum, we can only know the status of sensory experience in a partial and observer-biased fashion.

Proprioception

There is widespread agreement about the biologic import of joint position sense. Information from muscle tendons and joint capsules is faithfully relayed to the thalamus and cortex, and parallel information (including the muscle spindles) goes to the cerebellum. Receptors in the joint capsule fire in relation to joint angle, while pressure receptors in skin and subcutaneous tissue reflect physical forces on the body wall. This detailed information enables the brain to make a complete reconstruction of the position of the head, trunk, and limbs in space. The CNS is aware of the current postural attitude, the weight of the elbow on the chair arm, and the fact that the shoes are perhaps too tight. We cannot even imagine the experience of somatosensory deprivation. The dorsal column pathway also maintains a detailed map of the body wall for tactile discrimination. This includes information for localizing touch, and impulses from receptors surrounding hair follicles.

Organization of the Dorsal Column Pathway

Large-fiber afferents whose cell bodies lie in the dorsal root ganglia enter the dorsal horn, pass medially, and ascend without synapse in the posterior column pathway. The first synapse is in the medulla, in the dorsal column nuclei. Second-order neurons cross the medulla as the internal arcuate fibers to ascend via the medial lemniscus to the thalamus. A specific thalamocortical projection to S1 and SII somatosensory cortex preserves a precise somatotopic map of the contralateral trunk and limbs.

The dorsal column pathway and the anterolateral system are contrasted in Figure 4-10. Several important organizational differences are evident. Pain afferents make their first synapse in the dorsal horn;

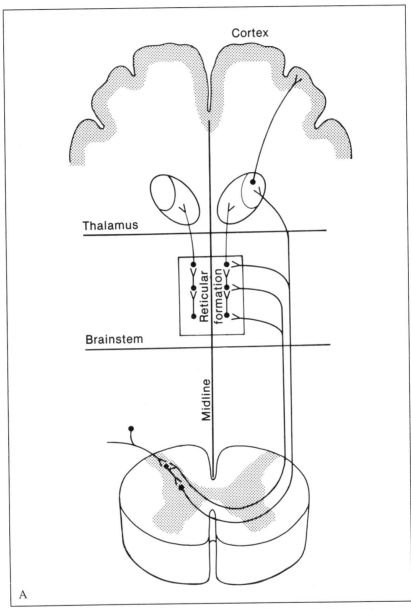

FIGURE 4-10. Schematic flow diagrams contrast the organization of the anterolateral spinothalamic tract with the dorsal column pathway. The anterolateral system crosses the midline near its origin, and has some bilateral representation. A large subset terminates in the brainstem recticular formation. The dorsal column pathway ascends uncrossed, and is more coherent. (Adapted from E.R. Kandel and J.H. Schwartz [eds.], *Principles of Neural Science* [2nd ed.]. New York: Elsevier, 1985, p. 183, with permission.)

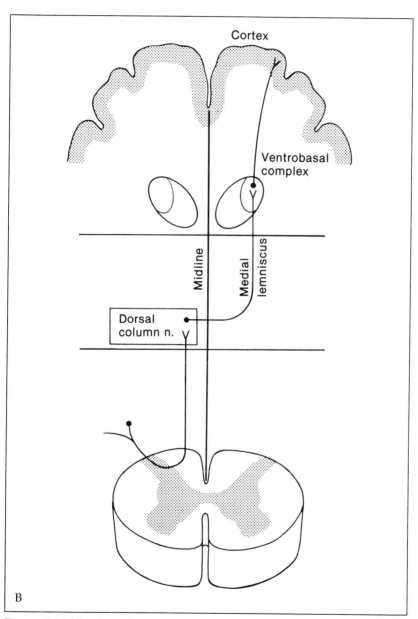

FIGURE 4-10 (Continued).

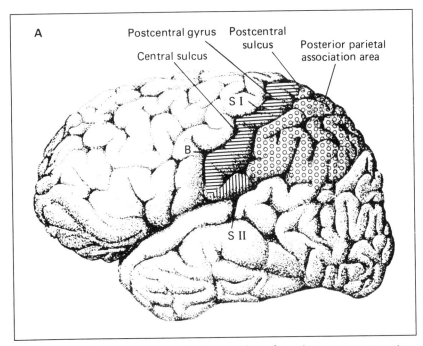

FIGURE 4-11. Somatosensory cortical areas: SI is the primary sensory cortex (Brodmann's areas 1, 2, and 3). SII is an accessory sensory cortex. The adjacent portion of the parietal lobe is sensory association cortex. (From E.R. Kandel and J.H. Schwartz [eds.], *Principles of Neural Science* [2nd ed.]. New York: Elsevier, 1985, p. 181, with permission.)

second- and third-order neurons cross the midline in the spinal cord prior to ascent. Proprioceptive afferents do not make an initial synapse in the spinal cord; they ascend ipsilaterally. The dorsal column pathway is somatotopically organized, and tightly focused spatially. Cells in the brainstem and thalamic relay nuclei display small and precise receptive fields. By contrast, the anterolateral system is diffuse. The projection to the reticular formation is not topographically organized. A subset of the anterolateral system remains uncrossed, so there is bilateral representation of pain afferents. By contrast with the engineering of the dorsal column pathway, the anterolateral pathway is a sloppy system. It recruits a wide response from subcortical structures, but high-level resolution is poor for discrimination and localization.

Cortical Representation of Somatic Sensation

Two segments of cerebral cortex in each hemisphere are specialized for processing somatic sensory information. The primary sensory cortex

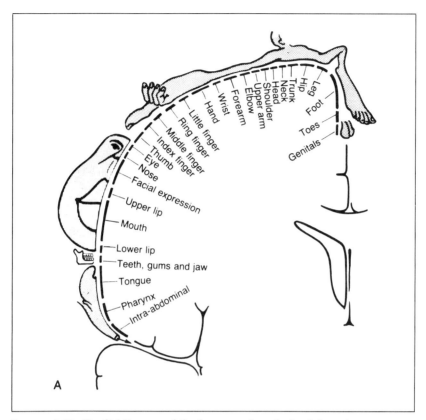

FIGURE 4-12. Penfield's map of the homunculus, derived from intraoperative stimulation of the cerebral cortex. Separate topographic mappings are depicted for primary sensory (A) and motor cortex (B). (Adapted from W. Penfield and T. Rasmussen, *The Cerebral Cortex of Man: A Clinical Study of Localization of Function*. New York: Macmillan, 1950, p. 373, with permission.)

cortex (SI) is located in the postcentral gyrus. SI includes Brodmann's areas 1, 2, and 3. Inputs to SI are somatotopically organized and represent exclusively the contralateral body. Secondary sensory cortex (SII) receives its own set of thalamocortical afferents, which are to some degree bilateral. SII is located in the parietal lobe immediately above the sylvian fissure; somewhat less is known about its function (Fig. 4-11). Posterior to area SI is the sensory association cortex and the higher-order association cortex of the posterior parietal lobe. The latter synthesizes multimodal sensory information about the contralateral body wall and its relationships within extrapersonal space.

Early studies on the physiology of sensory cortex revealed a precise representational map of the contralateral body wall and limbs onto cortical field SI. Marshal and Woolsey discovered this organizational

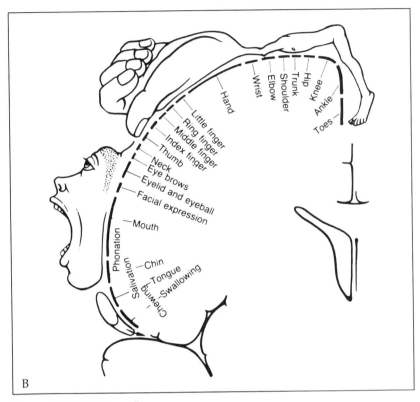

FIGURE 4-12 (Continued).

pattern of sensory cortex in the 1930s while exploring the cortical activity evoked by cutaneous stimuli in laboratory animals. Penfield was able to stimulate the human cortex directly in patients undergoing epilepsy surgery under light anesthesia. When cortex in SI was stimulated, the patients reported a tactile sensation on the corresponding part of the contralateral body. The topography of the cortical sensory map could thus be studied and reconstructed. Figure 4-12 was derived in this fashion from Penfield's intraoperative studies. Jacksonian seizures sometimes propagate along a path defined by the cortical map.

This representation of the body surface on the cortical mantle is known as the "homunculus." A separate homunculus for the body is situated in the primary motor cortex. The homunculus in the brain is an odd and rather distorted image. The caricature depicted is an internal representation that respects neighborhood relationships, but assigns space in proportion to sensory innervation density. The lips, tongue, and fingers are a rich source of sense experience for man.

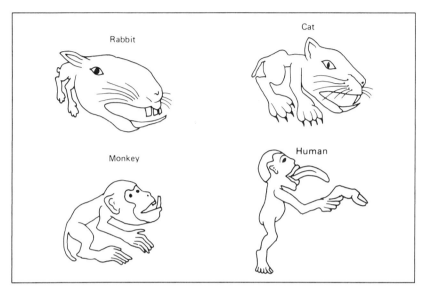

FIGURE 4-13. Reconstruction of cortical sensory representation in four species. The caricatures depict the amount of cortical space given to respective body parts. (From E.R. Kandel and J.H. Schwartz [eds.], *Principles of Neural Science* [2nd ed.]. New York: Elsevier, 1985, p. 191, with permission.)

These regions are dense with cutaneous receptors, and they are allocated a disproportionately large space in the homunculus. Woolsey's comparative studies of the cortical map provide us with an insight into the sense experience of animals (Fig. 4-13). An enormous field in the cortex of the rat, for instance, is dedicated to the rows of whiskers on the face by which the rat explores his world. The space on the homunculus for human face hairs is quite small, but the lips, tongue, and fingers have grown to occupy an enormous share.

Extracellular recording from sensory cortex in animals has yielded further insights into the organization of somatic sensation. Each neuron in a sensory cortex such as SI has a receptive field: that area within the space of sensory experience from which stimulation excites (or inhibits) cell firing. The size of the receptive field varies in inverse relation to innervation density. Tiny receptive fields in the representation of the fingertips reflect the exquisitely fine-grained sensory capability of this region. A vertical column of SI neurons contains cells with virtually identical receptive fields. This column of nerve cells receives regional inhibition from neighboring columns. Activation of a cell column will thus evoke a wave of inhibition within an annulus of surrounding cortex. This pattern of *surround inhibition,* described first in the visual cortex, is hard-wired into the cortical architecture. This

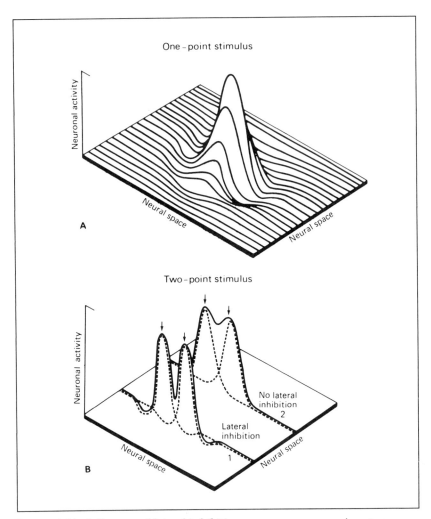

FIGURE 4-14. Influence of lateral inhibition on sensory processing: two-point discrimination. A. When a single point on the skin is stimulated, a pattern of cortical activation is evoked. B. The distribution of activation when two adjacent points are stimulated is depicted along one dimension. Without lateral inhibition, the images tend to fuse. (From E.R. Kandel and J.H. Schwartz [eds.], *Principles of Neural Science* [2nd ed.]. New York: Elsevier, 1985, p. 194, with permission.)

organization works to heighten the contrast in sensory processing, while limiting background noise. The representation of sense experience within a neighborhood of the column provides the substrate for interpreted sensory modalities, such as two-point discrimination (Fig. 4-14).

Interpreted (or Cortical) Sensory Modalities

The cerebral cortex, as mentioned above, can analyze the sense experience to produce complex perceptions. Most cortical neurons in SI show simple receptive fields of homogeneous type, specific for touch, pressure, or motion in joint capsules and tendons. A few, perhaps 5 to 10 percent, bear more complex receptive fields. Some such cells act as edge detectors, analogous to complex cells in the visual system, sensitive to the edge of an object, and perhaps its orientation. Others are direction-specific, firing only when a tactile sensation travels the body wall with a particular directional vector.

We have already seen how surround inhibition heightens contrast to facilitate *two-point discrimination*. The threshold for discrimination of two discrete pinpoint stimuli is a sensitive measure of density of innervation and its cortical representation and handling. The capacity for two-point discrimination is reduced when peripheral afferents are of poor quality (as in entrapment neuropathy), or in disease affecting SI cortex (such as stroke). The ability to read braille is perhaps man's highest accomplishment in tactile discrimination. Direction-sensitive cells in SI permit the analysis of sensation derived from moving stimuli. *Graphesthesia*, the ability to discern writing done onto the skin, is dependent on direction-sensitive cells to help us reconstruct the trace. *Stereognosis* is the capacity to discriminate objects placed in the hand. It is an interpreted sense experience dependent on the processing outlined above, most particularly on edge receptors. Stereognosis, two-point discrimination, and graphesthesia are often examined together as tests of sensory cortex facility. The ability to discern simultaneous tactile stimuli in remote parts of the body is used as a test of sensory association cortex in the parietal lobe.

Clinical Deficits: Localizing the Pattern of Sensory Loss

Neurologic injury to sensory structures results in symptoms and signs, positive and negative phenomena. Negative phenomena are experienced as the absence of a particular class of sensation: analgesia (the absence of pain), anesthesia (the total absence of sensation). Equally important are intrusive positive phenomena, such as pain and paresthesias, the asleep numbness which often accompanies peripheral nervous system disease. The first step in neurologic diagnosis is anatomic localization, and localization can often be inferred from the pattern of sensory abnormality.

Diseases of peripheral nerve may affect all modalities, or may be selective for nerve fibers of particular size or physiologic class (i.e., diameter, myelination). Localization will be evident in the distribution of sensory loss, which should conform to the territory of a peripheral nerve. Burning pain, irritating paresthesia, and cutaneous hypersensitivity (hyperpathia) are often described in patients with nerve injuries. In proximal nerve injuries, autonomic change may be prominent. Generalized neuropathies cause sensory loss in a distal "stocking-and-glove" distribution.

Nerve root lesions, such as occur with degenerative arthritis or a herniated intervertebral disc, are characterized by a lancinating pain which radiates out of the involved dermatome. Associated features may include numbness or paresthesia; often a sense of coldness is described with the pain. Radicular pains are often aggravated by cough, straining at stool, or Valsalva maneuvers which transmit pressure down the spinal subarachnoid space. Positive phenomena, especially pain, may be evoked by positions which stretch the nerve root, such as rotation of the neck or straight leg raising.

Spinal syndromes display sensory change in relation to the topography of the injury. In hemisection of the spinal cord (Brown-Séquard syndrome), there is ipsilateral paralysis, with loss of joint position and vibration sense below the lesion. A band of complete analgesia may be seen at the involved segment, with contralateral analgesia below. In diseases of the central zone of the cord (syringomyelia or anterior spinal artery territory infarction), there is generally injury to anterior horn cells. An important clue in these cases is *dissociated sensory loss*, which may be restricted to the involved segments. Pain and temperature, whose second-order neurons cross in the anterior white commissure, may be lost in the involved dermatomes, while joint position and vibration sense are preserved. If and when the lesion enlarges and the anterolateral tract becomes involved, sacral sparing is sometimes observed. (Sacral fibers are outermost in the tract.)

Cortical lesions commonly spare pain sensation, and pain should not intrude as a positive phenomenon. Focal sensory seizures may cause transient paresthetic sensations, which are usually not painful. The characteristic feature of damage to sensory cortical areas is the loss of interpreted sensation: two-point discrimination, graphesthesia, stereognosis. Touch localization may be quite impaired. In addition, patients with parietal lobe disease will show extinction: the inattention to stimulation of the contralateral side when simultaneous stimulation is provided on the normal side. Neglect may be a phenomenon with right parietal disease (see Chap. 8).

Somatosensory cortical evoked potentials are sometimes used to explore for subtle demyelinating injury to sensory pathways. These tests are also available for auditory and visual systems, and have a wide clinical usefulness.

The Deafferentated Limb

Great clumsiness is sometimes observed in a limb after a loss of somatosensory afferents. Sherrington observed that monkeys that had surgical deafferentation of a limb failed to use the limb at all for purposeful movements. Human patients affected by tabetic neurosyphilis, common prior to the widespread availability of penicillin, were observed to suffer radicular (root entry zone) pains and a clumsy deafferentation disorder of gait. The question raised by these observations concerns the reliance of motor performance on sensory feedback. What is the impact on skilled motor acts of a loss of afferent sensory information?

Detailed studies have come from the primate work of Taub, and more recently from the clinical observations of Rothwell, Marsden, et al. These investigators studied motor performance in an unfortunate patient with deafferentation of the limbs due to severe neuropathy. Many motor skills were preserved. The patient was able to imitate a wide variety of manual movements with rapidity and grace. He was also able to perform a number of prelearned motor skills, despite loss of sensation and the absence of direct visual control. Despite his facility in the laboratory, this same patient found his hands relatively useless for a variety of fine tasks important in daily life. Holding an egg without breaking it requires constant sensory monitoring; fastening buttons and writing were almost impossible for this patient.

Investigators have suggested that complex motor tasks can often be performed without ongoing sensory feedback, by virtue of a prelearned set of motor instructions. Somatosensory feedback is thought to be more important in the difficult process of acquisition and refinement of motor skills. Mastering a tennis serve, learning to ride a bicycle, learning to eat with chopsticks—these are tasks learned by trial and error in which somatosensory feedback is more crucial. Taub's monkeys and Marsden's patient were able to learn new motor skills with the aid of considerable direct visual guidance, but the learning of some new skills was impaired. Marsden's patient, for instance, bought a new car; but he found that he was unable to operate the gearshift, and ultimately had to give it up. Such studies provide a more sophisticated understanding of the dependence of motor performance on afferent sensory information.

The Phantom Limb

In patients suffering traumatic amputation of a limb, persistent and bothersome sense experience may be reported localized to the absent

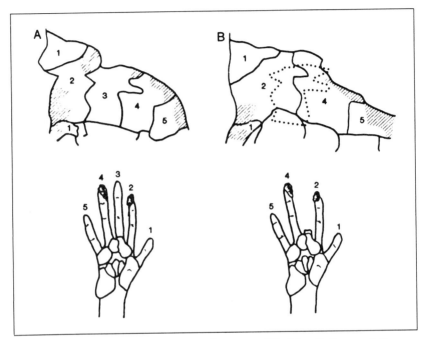

FIGURE 4-15. Cortical map in the monkey is modified by digit amputation. A. The cortical map of the hand prior to amputation of digit 3, as derived by microelectrode recording during tactile stimulation. B. Several weeks after amputation, an orderly shift of the cortical mapping is observed. (From M. Merzenich et al., Somatosensory cortical map changes after digit amputation in adult monkeys. *J. Comp. Neurol.* 224 : 591, 1984, with permission.)

extremity. Phantoms are sometimes perceived in an odd attitude and may be painful. Phantoms in amputee patients often recede over time, telescoping into vestigial limbs, or merely connected digits. It is typical for the imagined phantom to be distorted or bent in a painfully unphysiologic fashion—a position which may be a residual nervous system trace from the traumatic experience in which the limb was lost.

The loss of peripheral afferents leaves intact the cortical substrate for somatic sensation. The limb area on the homunculus persists when the physical body part for which it stands has been lost. Cortical processing continues in the absence of meaningful input, though some information of a dysfunctional sort may be generated from the proximal stump of the nerve. In order to rid the patient of his phantom, the corresponding piece of cortex would need to be silenced.

The prevailing view of cortical maps as internal representations of sensory space suggests that these relationships are indelibly hard-wired. Cortical afferent connections are established during development, and cortical columns are dedicated to a particular receptive field. Recent animal studies suggest that the plasticity of somatosensory cortex has been underestimated. Under certain circumstances, these internal maps retain the capacity for rearrangement. Merzenich and colleagues have demonstrated reorganization of the hand area of cortical field SI in the adult owl monkey after amputation of a digit. Over several weeks, the cortical field representing the missing digit, an area of some 1,200 μm, loses territory as the adjacent digital fields expand (Fig. 4-15). This research suggests that the homunculus may be the product of a dynamic synaptic architecture with some plasticity (the capacity for change in its connectivity relationships). The research gives us a new basis for understanding regressive changes in the phantom limb, as reported by some patients with the passage of time.

BIBLIOGRAPHY

Basbaum, A., and Fields, H. Endogenous pain control mechanisms: Review and hypothesis. *Ann. Neurol.* 4 : 451–462, 1978.

Fields, H.L. *Pain.* New York: McGraw-Hill, 1987.

Levine, J., Gordon, N., and Fields, H. The mechanism of placebo analgesia. *Lancet* 2 : 654–647, 1978.

Merzenich, M., et al. Somatosensory cortical map changes after digit amputation in adult monkeys. *J. Comp. Neurol.* 224 : 591, 1984.

Penfield, W., and Rasmussen, T. *The Cerebral Cortex of Man: A Clinical Study of Localization of Function.* New York: Macmillan, 1950.

Rothwell, J.D., et al. Manual motor performance in a deafferented man. *Brain* 105 : 515–542, 1982.

Snyder, S. Opiate receptors and internal opiates. *Sci. Am.* 236 : 44–56, 1977.

Wall, P.D. The gate control theory of pain. *Brain* 101 : 1–18, 1978.

CHAPTER 5

Disorders of Motor Control

The capacity for voluntary movement is essential to us in our daily activities. As mobile creatures who walk, speak, and manipulate tools, we rely on control over a small pool of specialized motor neurons in the ventral gray matter of the spinal cord and brainstem. These effector neurons translate our intentions into actions. Diseases of the nervous system can compromise control of movement, or render us paralyzed. To understand this vulnerability, it is necessary to consider first the production of normal voluntary movement.

BOTTOM-UP VIEW: THE MOTOR SYSTEM AS A COMPOSITION OF REFLEXES

The traditional view regards the motor system as a hierarchical organization. Lower centers are capable of a limited repertoire of responses, rather specialized and stereotyped. Successively higher centers deploy these "reflexes" in a more complex and flexible manner. Control is ultimately exercised from the top down in a rigid fashion, somewhat like the military chain of command.

The motor unit is the fundamental component in this scheme. All thoughts and instructions converge on a small pool of effector nerve cells, 2 to 3 million in number. Only through these neurons can the nervous system influence events in the outside world. Each alpha motor neuron receives roughly 10,000 synaptic contacts, competing to motivate its firing. In parallel, gamma efferents to skeletal muscle regulate the bias of stretch receptors in the muscle spindle.

Within the gray matter of the spinal cord, the alpha motor neuron is part of a local segmental network. The nucleus in the anterior horn organizes the graded recruitment of motor units and coordinates a variety of spinal reflexes. Muscle can be used to generate a gradually increasing force. Two principles govern the firing of motor neurons when the muscle contracts. More force can be achieved by increased

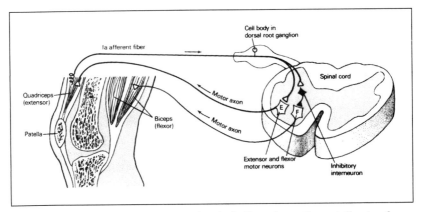

FIGURE 5-1. The monosynaptic tendon jerk: Stretch on the patellar tendon stimulates stretch receptors in the muscle spindle, and excites Ia afferents. Motor neuron fires, causing contraction and shortening of the quadriceps muscle. Reciprocal pattern of local inhibition causes relaxation of the antagonist muscle. (From E.R. Kandel and J.H. Schwartz [eds.], *Principles of Neural Science* [2nd ed.]. New York: Elsevier, 1985, p. 109, with permission.)

rate of firing (rate coding). Smaller motor units generate small forces, and are used first. As force increases, larger units are recruited in ascending order (the Henneman size principle). As a rule, muscles are organized in antagonist pairs, which oppose each other's action (e.g., biceps and triceps). Contraction of a muscle is associated with relaxation in the antagonist. The segmental mechanism arranges this reciprocal activation. Under some circumstances, fragments of complex walking or swimming movements can be evoked from the gray matter of the spinal cord. (Never underestimate the capabilities of the isolated spinal cord!)

Reflexes vary from the simple, monosynaptic tendon jerk to the more complex polysynaptic, multisegmental reflex which effects the automatic withdrawal of a limb from pain. The muscle spindle controls the tendon jerk (Fig. 5-1). When there is a sudden stretch on the muscle and its spindle, receptors in the intrafusal fiber excite Ia afferents to the gray matter of the spinal segment. The synapse from the Ia afferent is located so as to compel firing of the alpha motor neuron, causing the muscle to contract and shorten. Over the longer term, the spinal gray attempts to regulate muscle tone so as to match afferent signals generated by the spindle. Gamma efferents to the spindle adjust the gain, and increase the dynamic range of the stretch receptor. Withdrawal from pain is a more complex response, requiring coordinated activity over several segments of the spinal cord. Imagine that the patient steps on a tack (Fig. 5-2). Cutaneous sensory receptors

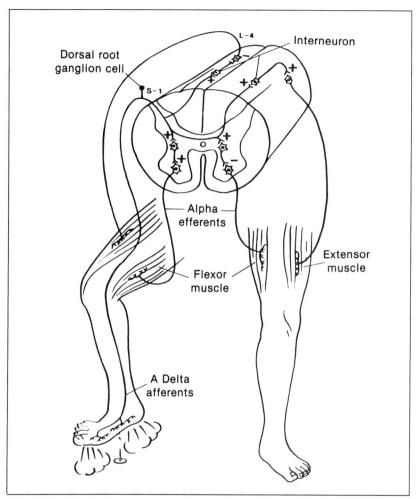

FIGURE 5-2. Withdrawal from pain: a multisynaptic and multisegmental reflex. Painful stimulus to the sole of the foot excites the flexor motor units on the right side from the anterior tibial (L5) up to the psoas (L1). Meanwhile, the contralateral extensors brace the left leg for the forces of reaction. (From J. Daube et al., *Medical Neurosciences* [2nd ed.]. Boston: Little, Brown, 1986, p. 313, with permission.)

trigger the pain pathway, including the posterior gray matter of the spinal cord (substantia gelatinosa) at S1. Impulses are relayed over the local (propriospinal) tract to coordinate the contraction of the anterior tibial muscles (L5), the hamstrings (L5) and the psoas muscle (L1–2) to withdraw the leg. At the appropriate moment, tone is increased in the contralateral extensors to brace the opposite limb for the forces of reaction.

Descending influences on the spinal segment and motor pool include the vestibulospinal, rubrospinal, reticulospinal, and corticospinal tracts. The vestibular nuclei and vestibulospinal tract effect postural supporting responses, often called "righting reflexes" in the older literature. If we lacked these automatic postural responses, we would be unable to stand while riding a bus or streetcar. (If the bus were to brake unexpectedly, standing passengers would fall over like so many carved wooden figurines.) Response in the limbs to vestibular stimulation or a change in support-surface afferents often has an extensor bias. Its influence is partly balanced by the rubrospinal tract, which has a flexor bias. The vestibulospinal tract is the substrate for decerebrate posture. In patients with extensive injury to the forebrain, with loss of the corticospinal and rubrospinal tracts, the vestibulospinal tract may be the dominant motor pathway. Such patients, usually comatose, respond to head movement or noxious stimuli by tonic extensor posturing in the neck and limbs.

The reticulospinal tract is a more diffuse anatomic system, consisting of spinal efferents from the brainstem reticular nuclei. It has a medial and a lateral division. The medial segment carries motor instructions for voiding the urinary bladder, and for control of respirations. Autonomic cardiovascular reflexes are also influenced by the reticulospinal system.

The corticospinal tract is the main pathway for cerebral control of movement. Thirty percent of the pathway originates in the large pyramidal cells of the motor cortex (Brodmann's area 4). The rest is from adjacent cortical fields. This pathway is often referred to as the *pyramidal tract*. Twenty percent of the fibers in the tract enjoy direct synapse on alpha motor neurons in the spinal cord of man, giving the pathway unrestricted access to the motor unit. In most animals, corticospinal instructions are processed in the anterior horn, but in man the corticospinal tract tyrannizes the motor pool. It brings finesse and speed to movement. Most heavily innervated are distal muscles of the upper extremity. The corticospinal pathway enables fractionation of hand movements, required in fine motor tasks (such as buttoning, typing, piano playing). Experiments in the primate by Lawrence and Kuypers demonstrate the specialized function of this pathway. Unlike humans with large pyramidal lesions, monkeys are able to recover the ability to ambulate and use the arms after section of this tract. They are permanently unable to pick food pellets out of a recessed dish, a task requiring fractionated movements and opposition of the digits.

At the next level of organization, the motor system has remained an enigma. The basal ganglia and cerebellum are involved in the control of movement, but the complexity of these structures has obscured their exact role. Lesions in this part of the nervous system produce a disorder of posture, gait, and motor control, yet the normal function is not understood at a cellular level. The information that converges on the motor cortex and the processing which goes on there is likewise poorly understood.

TOP-DOWN ANALYSIS: THE ROBOTIC PERSPECTIVE

Another approach to the problem of motor control adopts the perspective of the systems engineer. We examine the capabilities of the motor system through its behavioral repertoire. What happens in the central nervous system (CNS) in preparation for movement? What problems must the nervous system solve in organizing each performance?

Figure 5-3 shows a computed average of electroencephalographic (EEG) activity in the 2 seconds surrounding a voluntary movement. The computer can average hundreds of events, such that the extraneous background activity averages out. A focused potential is observed over the motor cortex 60 to 100 msec prior to the muscle twitch, representing the firing of the corticospinal tract. If you look at the trace in the moments prior, you will observe a slowly rising potential, somewhat diffuse, over central areas. This readiness potential (*Bereitschafts-potential*) begins 500 msec in anticipation of the movement. In the realm of cellular neurophysiology, half a second is a very long time. This electrical event marks the first step in planning for the subsequent movement.

The schematic diagram from Allen and Tsukahara (Fig. 5-4) represents a hypothesis about the events in this half second. The will to move impacts on the association cortex of the frontal and parietal lobes. This formulation does not propose to solve the mind-body problem, but rather indicates the first neural representation of the intention to move. A goal for the movement is then fed forward to the basal ganglia and cerebellum, to elaborate a set of detailed instructions. The lateral cerebellum, according to this hypothesis, contributes information on muscle burst duration and timing. The basal ganglia contribute learned, preprogrammed subroutines, and help shape and initiate movement. The detailed plan is then passed to the motor cortex, which fires the corticospinal tract to execute. Recall that this is not a computational model for these events, but rather a crude hypothesis about the organization of movement.

A useful concept in neurophysiology is that of the motor program. We believe the nervous system stores and elaborates a high-level specification for most learned movement. Specific details regarding individual muscles are determined at the time of execution. The notion

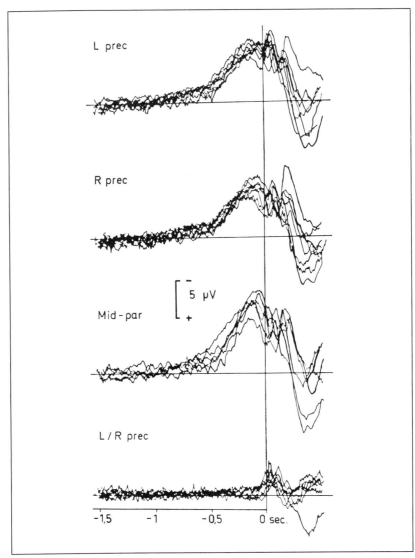

FIGURE 5-3. The readiness potential: In anticipation of a rehearsed voluntary movement of the index finger, a slowly rising negative potential is recorded from the scalp. The potentials are obtained by back-averaging of repeated events. Eight experiments were done on different days with the same subject; each trace represents about 1,000 movements per experiment. The readiness potential (*Bereitschaftspotential*) can be observed in recordings from left (L) and right (R) precentral (prec) and midparietal (Mid-par) regions 500 to 800 msec before the onset of movement (time 0). (From L. Deecke, P. Scheid, and H.H. Kornhuber, Distribution of readiness potential, pre-motion positivity, and motor potential of the human cerebral cortex preceding voluntary finger movements. *Exp. Brain Res.* 7 : 158–168, 1969, with permission.)

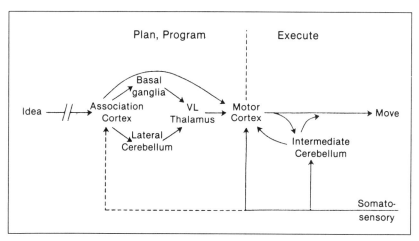

FIGURE 5-4. Diagram depicts a hypothesis about the organization of voluntary movement. The will to move (IDEA) impacts on association cortex, which activates motor cortex with the help of the basal ganglia and lateral cerebellum. Execution of ongoing movement includes some refinement via the intermediate zone of the cerebellum. (From J. Eccles, *The Understanding of the Brain* [2nd ed.]. New York: McGraw-Hill, 1976, p. 136, with permission.)

of preprogrammed "chunks" of movement is appealing, as there is really no time for online sensory feedback and course correction. A skilled typist, or a pianist playing a Chopin nocturne may produce 10 or more finger movements in a second! By the time somatosensory feedback is processed at higher levels of the nervous system, several additional movements have already occurred. A good typist will commonly become aware of an error one or two words back. Skilled movements of this nature are probably highly programmed and done in an "open loop" fashion, without much reliance on sensory feedback. Feedback is likely to be more important in motor learning, and in other tasks which specifically require sensory guidance and precision control. The process of motor program acquisition is a slow and effortful one, as anyone can attest who has struggled to learn a tennis serve or master the use of chopsticks. Experts on the subject of motor control believe that the basal ganglia are responsible for the elaboration and automatic execution of learned motor plans, details of which are programmed with the cerebellum according to the environment at run time.

The anatomic substrate for this processing in the basal ganglia is the striatal loop, shown in Figure 5-5. To trace the connections, begin at the neostriatum (the caudate and putamen). (We neglect for the moment connections with the substantia nigra.) The principal afferents

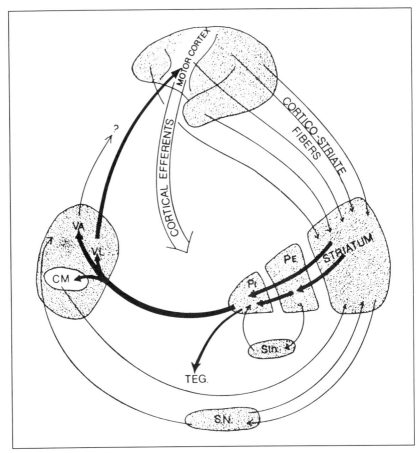

FIGURE 5-5. The striatal loop: major afferent and efferent connections of the basal ganglia. Striatal afferents come from the cerebral cortex, centromedian (CM) and intralaminar thalamic nuclei, and substantia nigra (SN). Globus pallidus, external (PE) and internal divisions (PI), project to the subthalamic nucleus (Stn), midbrain tegmentum (TEG.), and motor thalamus. Thalamocortical projections to premotor cortex, principally M2, complete the loop. (From M. DeLong, Basal Ganglia, Unit Activity During Movement. In F.O. Schmidt and F.G. Worden [eds.], *The Neurosciences, Third Study Program.* Cambridge, Mass.: MIT Press, 1974, p. 320, with permission.)

to this structure derive from the neocortex, in a large ordered mapping. The corticostriate projection is thought to utilize the excitatory amino acid glutamate as its principal transmitter. The efferents from the caudate and putamen funnel through the globus pallidus. The striatopallidal outflow has three parts: A branch division innervates the subthalamic nucleus. A second division goes to the tegmental area in the midbrain. The third and principal outflow is to the ventro-lateral thalamus. This thalamic nucleus projects to motor cortical structures, principally the supplementary motor cortex (M2), to complete the loop. The striatal loop is the major re-entrant pathway of the basal ganglia. By analogy to computer programming, where much of importance happens in a loop, some experts believe the striatal loop is a key pathway for motor programming. Penny and Young propose that the striatal loop maintains ongoing movements, selects new movement, and suppresses unwanted movements.

Motor instructions are ultimately compiled and executed in the motor cortex. The corticospinal tract is the principal effector pathway. Evarts, Fetz, and others have demonstrated that the upper motor neurons control the force generated by limb muscles during a movement. The frequency of firing in area 4 neurons encodes the muscle force, rather than explicitly representing the position of the limb. Bizzi has also studied the cells of the motor cortex in awake, behaving animals. His research suggests that cortical motor neurons encode a field of elastic forces, which in turn specify the postural attitude of the limb in space. These forces may determine the trajectory for movement.

THE UPPER MOTOR NEURON SYNDROME

The upper motor neuron syndrome is the most common motor control disorder in clinical practice. The four principal characteristics are paralysis, hyperreflexia, increased muscle tone, and the sign of Babinski. The effects are often attributed to loss of the corticospinal tract, though other descending pathways may be responsible for aspects of the clinical syndrome. (Pure lesions of the corticospinal pathway in man result in flaccid paralysis.) Weakness may be partial, or there may be complete paralysis and inability to make a movement at will. Control over the distal limbs and the extensor muscles is most severely compromised.

Spasticity denotes an increase in stretch reflexes and a state of increased tone, palpable during active or passive movement. Activity is increased in both alpha and gamma (spindle) efferents, due to a change in spinal interneuron modulation of motor neurons. The "clasp-knife" phenomenon is often observed: a stiff initial resistance that gives way as the Golgi tendon organ overrides the muscle spindle. Release from spinal control results in overactivity of stretch reflexes, and a change in the activity of flexor reflex afferents which mediate cutaneous reflexes. The Babinski sign is a special case. In the absence of descending modulation, the spinal motor pool is widely activated when the sole of the foot is scratched. The result is extension of the great toe, abduction of the other digits, and fragments of the withdrawal reflex.

While spasticity can be disabling, most patients are more troubled by the loss of control and dexterity. Like Lawrence and Kuypers' monkeys, patients are unable to fractionate distal movements. The upper extremity may be able to generate a powerful flexor movement and grasp, but movement is slow and the postural attitude of the limb is unnatural.

PARKINSON'S DISEASE

First described by James Parkinson in 1817, Parkinson's disease is a common malady in older people. Prevalence is about 1.5 percent in the population over 65. Patients complain of stiffness and slowness at daily activities. Parkinson's disease is distinguished by four cardinal clinical manifestations: bradykinesia, rigidity, tremor, and a characteristic disorder of posture and gait. *Bradykinesia* describes the slowness, the viscosity, the difficulty experienced when producing voluntary movement on demand. *Rigidity* is uniform through the range of movement, and is commonly associated with a 3- to 5-cps *tremor at rest*. A flexed attitude predominates in posture. Patients often display loss of balance (postural instability) and a characteristic *shuffling gait*. Associated features include dysarthria, poverty of facial expression, tiny, illegible handwriting (micrographia), and a general disorder of motor program execution. Freezing occurs during ongoing movement, patients have difficulty doing two things at once, and great difficulty may be encountered in initiating movement.

Pathology shows loss of pigmented neurons in the pars compacta of the substantia nigra, a pallor in the midbrain that can often be appreciated grossly (Fig. 5-6). Nigral neurons are a specialized population of nerve cells that contain neuromelanin and manufacture the neurotransmitter dopamine. There are 500,000 dopamine neurons in the young adult brain, most of which are in the midbrain substantia nigra and adjacent ventral tegmental area. Dopamine neurons in the nigra and other catecholamine neurons in the brainstem are selectively lost in Parkinson's disease. Intraneuronal inclusion bodies (Lewy bodies) are seen in some of the remaining pigmented neurons when these areas are examined microscopically. These inclusions are a biologic marker for the disease process.

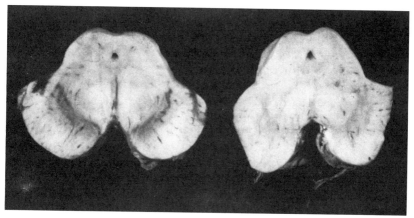

FIGURE 5-6. Comparison of midbrain from patient with Parkinson's disease (*left*) and normal (*right*) shows depigmentation of the substantia nigra. This is due to a loss of dopamine neurons, which contain neuromelanin. (From Dr. James Morris, Brigham and Womens Hospital, Boston.)

Basis for Bradykinesia and Rigidity

What does the substantia nigra have to do with the basal ganglia and the control of movement? Nigral neurons are the source of the dopaminergic projection to the striatum (the caudate and putamen). A parallel pathway projects from the ventral tegmental area to the frontal cortex and limbic structures (the mesocortical and mesolimbic dopamine system). The nigrostriatal projection is the largest of these, and is highly *divergent:* one nigral neuron may contact 100,000 cells in the striatum. Current studies suggest that dopamine is inhibitory at some striatal receptors, but may be excitatory at others. Many of the nerve terminals release dopamine at nonclassic or en passage synapses, suffusing the striatum with neurotransmitter. The anatomy suggests a modulatory role for nigral afferents to the basal ganglia, rather than a precise information system. The implication is that the substantia nigra acts as a control point, to regulate the flow of process in the striatal loop (much like the choke or microprocessor control on an automobile carburetor). Loss of nigral neurons in Parkinson's disease produces depletion of dopamine in the striatum. There is a large functional reserve in the system, such that 50 to 70 percent of the striatal dopamine content can be lost without clinical effect. Past this threshold, loss of dopaminergic innervation causes a disturbance of normal striatopallidal activity: a syndrome of bradykinesia, rigidity, and difficulty at execution of planned movement.

TABLE 5-1. Differential Diagnosis of Parkinsonism

Idiopathic Parkinson's disease
Postencephalitic parkinsonism
Drug-induced parkinsonism
Stroke (especially lacunar strokes in the basal ganglia)
Systems degenerations
   Shy-Drager syndrome
   Progressive supranuclear palsy
   Striatonigral degeneration
   Olivopontocerebellar atrophy
Alzheimer's disease with extrapyramidal rigidity
Trauma, midbrain injury
Tumor, vascular malformation
Chemical intoxication
  Manganese
  Carbon monoxide
  MPTP

New Ideas on the Cause of Parkinson's Disease

Parkinson's disease is a progressive disorder. Loss of nigral neurons is gradual, and most likely begins years before clinical symptoms are evident. The condition is not inherited. The cause of cell death in Parkinson's disease has not yet been identified, though viruses, toxins, and a number of other diseases can cause parkinsonian manifestations (Table 5-1). Such causes account for roughly 15 percent of patients presenting clinically with a parkinsonian syndrome. The rest of the cases are called "idiopathic."

An interesting clue was provided by a miniepidemic of a parkinsonian syndrome among young drug abusers in California in the 1970s. Parkinson's disease is characteristically a disorder of older people (onset under age 40 is unusual). So it was a surprise when Langston and others first encountered a cluster of cases in young people. All had been exposed to methylphenyltetrahydropyridine (MPTP), a byproduct in the synthesis of "designer drugs" (chemically altered versions of controlled substances). The patients looked like they had Parkinson's disease, and their symptoms improved dramatically when they were treated with levodopa. Animal studies confirm that the toxin MPTP destroys nigral neurons. A primate model exhibits a parkinsonian syndrome with eosinophilic inclusions in the substantia nigra. The neurotoxin is specific for the same class of neurons which are affected in human Parkinson's disease.

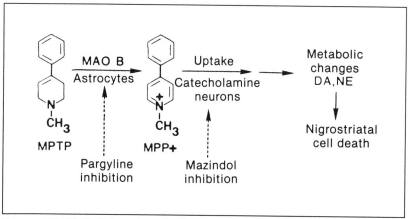

FIGURE 5-7. Methylphenyltetrahydropyridine (MPTP, *left*) requires oxidation to transform it into an active, toxic metabolite. In order to promote cell killing, a second step is necessary. Catecholamine uptake systems transport the toxin into the cell's metabolic machinery. Monoamine oxidase (MAO) inhibitors and antagonists of catecholamine uptake block the cytotoxic effect. DA = dopamine; NE = norepinephrine. (From S.H. Snyder and R.J. D'Amato, MPTP: A neurotoxin relevant to the pathophysiology of Parkinson's disease. *Neurology* 36 : 250–258, 1986, with permission.)

MPTP is not toxic to catecholamine neurons by itself, but requires oxidation to an active metabolite (Fig. 5-7). The oxidation of MPTP to its active form is handled in nervous tissues by monoamine oxidase, an enzyme present in the substantia nigra and basal ganglia, but not in the cell bodies of nigral neurons. The activated toxin is a substrate for the dopamine uptake mechanism in the nerve terminals. Once inside the nigral neurons, the activated toxin causes cell death. Inhibitors of monoamine oxidase B and inhibitors of high-affinity dopamine uptake protect against the toxicity of MPTP in primates.

This observation led Langston and Calne to propose a hypothesis about the cause of idiopathic Parkinson's disease. Nigral dopamine neurons undergo attrition in normal aging, at a rate of 8 to 9 percent per decade after age 60. Perhaps an environmental toxin causes loss of 50 to 60 percent of this cell population at some point during young adult life, an event which would not be associated with any immediate clinical manifestations. Symptoms and signs of Parkinson's disease might emerge 20 or 30 years later, as the loss of dopamine cells exceeds the critical threshold. Failure to defend against endogenous oxidant by-products of catecholamine metabolism might have the same end result. The specific chemical vulnerability of nigral neurons is now under active study in the hope that the cell biology of Parkinson's disease can be understood and altered.

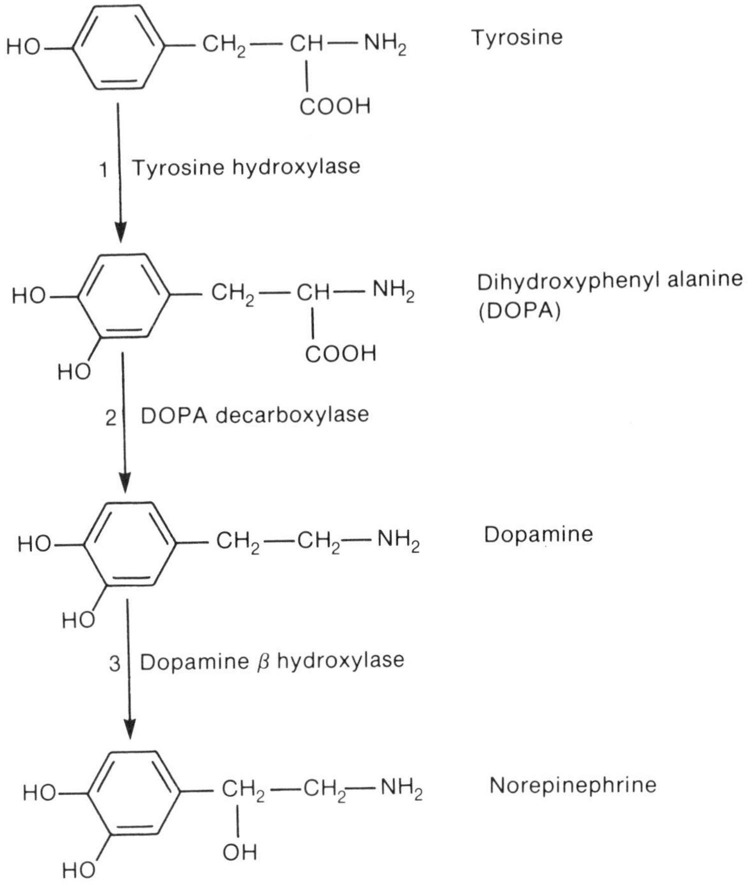

FIGURE 5-8. Biosynthesis of catecholamines dopamine and norepinephrine is summarized. Tyrosine hydroxylase reaction (1) is the rate-limiting step, and is normally under feedback control.

Dopamine Replacement Therapy

Therapy in Parkinson's disease is directed at replacement of dopamine in the CNS. The most commonly used treatment is dopamine replacement by *oral precursor loading*. The synthesis of neurotransmitter dopamine is reviewed in Fig. 5-8. Dopamine itself would not be a useful agent for pharmacotherapy; oral absorbtion is poor and it does not penetrate the blood-brain barrier. Systemically administered dopamine also has side effects in the (peripheral) autonomic nervous system, particularly a pressor effect on the cardiovascular system. The synthesis of catecholamines is regulated by tyrosine hydroxylase, the rate-limiting step in dopamine production. Orally administered levodopa is readily absorbed, and gains entrance into the brain in competition with other neutral amino acids. Bypassing the regulatory step, levodopa is freely converted to active dopamine in the nervous system, for storage and release at nerve terminals. Levodopa is commonly administered with a peripherally acting dopa decarboxylase inhibitor, in order to reduce the unwanted synthesis of catecholamines outside the nervous system.

Why does an increase in brain dopamine content affect the synaptic release of neurotransmitter? Under normal circumstances, an increase in brain dopamine content would not be expected to influence synaptic function. (The family car, after all, functions as well with a full tank of gas as with half a tank!) In Parkinson's disease, the few remaining dopamine neurons overfunction to compensate for the loss of others. Presumably they are limited in their effectiveness by the unavailability of transmitter; they are constantly running on empty. Only in these unusual circumstances would orally administered precursor be expected to make a difference.

With time, levodopa therapy becomes less satisfactory, due to progression of the disease, diminished capacity of the nigral system, and postsynaptic receptor changes in the striatum. Another treatment strategy is the use of direct-acting dopamine agonist drugs. These drugs act on the postsynaptic dopamine receptor, and do not rely on the nigral neuron for their effect. Unfortunately, existing drugs are somewhat less effective for most patients than levodopa. Anticholinergic drugs reduce rigidity and tremor somewhat, as acetylcholine and dopamine tend to have opposed effects in the striatum. A novel approach to dopamine replacement utilizes the transplantation of dopamine-producing tissues. In animal models, it is possible to place fetal substantia nigra tissue into the denervated striatum. Implanted cells sprout locally and establish new, functional synaptic contacts. (This approach is possible because the substantia nigra is a modulator, and imprecise reinnervation is tolerated. It is difficult to imagine this approach working as well for the spinal cord.) Human studies have used the patient's own adrenal medulla as an implant, with some modest success in a few cases. The protected status of the CNS may permit fetal substantia nigra grafts.

HUNTINGTON'S DISEASE

With Parkinson's disease, our understanding has allowed us to move from the realm of clinical phenomena to the synapse, and even beyond

TABLE 5-2. Differential Diagnosis of Choreic Disorders

Huntington's disease
Acute rheumatic chorea (Sydenham's)
Chorea gravidarum
Systemic lupus erythematosus
Chorea-acanthocytosis
Glutaric acidemia
Methylmalonic aciduria
Familial calcification of the basal ganglia
Acute vascular hemichorea
Senile chorea
Spontaneous oral dyskinesia in the edentulous patient
Drug-induced dyskinesias
    Levodopa, bromocriptine
    Anticholinergics
    Antihistamines
    Oral contraceptives
    Neuroleptics

to the molecular level. With the hyperkinetic movement disorders, we are not so knowledgeable. Chorea and the chorea-like dyskinesias provide a more typical example for study. Chorea is an older, descriptive term, which refers to rapid, irregular involuntary movements, sometimes associated with a dancing gait. A list of seemingly unrelated disorders can cause choreic movements (Table 5-2). All involve the basal ganglia, and presumably some final common pathway with regard to mechanism, though the details are not known. The archetype is the chorea of Huntington's disease.

The disease was described by George Huntington, an American physician, in 1872. He and his father observed the disorder among families of English descent living in the Hamptons (Long Island, New York). Careful genetic studies of known cases in the United States, South Africa, New Zealand, and Venezuela suggest a common ancestry in northern Europe. The disease was brought to North America by pilgrims from Bures, England in the 1640s.

Huntington's disease is a dominantly inherited disorder, characterized by dementia, chorea, and a behavioral disturbance. Depression is a common early feature, though many patients are described as loners and "difficult to get along with." Onset is in mid-adult life, when many patients have already had children. The average reproductive index is increased for Huntington's patients. Using restricted fragment polymorphisms and other gene mapping techniques, the genetic defect has been localized to the short arm of chromosome 4. The abnormal gene product has not yet been identified, nor is the mechanism known

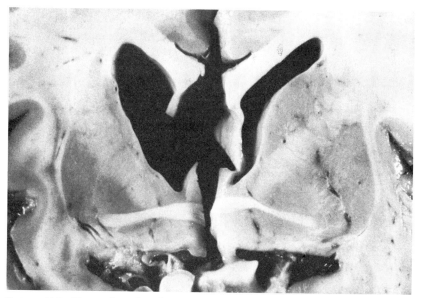

FIGURE 5-9. Coronal section from a patient with Huntington's disease (*left*) and normal control (*right*). Dilation of the lateral ventricle is due to gross atrophy of the caudate and putamen. (From Dr. James Morris, Brigham and Womens Hospital, Boston.)

for nervous tissue injury. The genetic abnormality somehow results in a selective loss of nerve cells with onset in adult life.

The movement disorder typically starts in the late thirties or early forties with facial twitch and irregular, piano-playing movements in the hands. With the passage of years, movements spread to the trunk and the characteristic erratic gait develops. After 15 to 20 years, patients often exhibit less chorea, and more rigidity and dystonia. Difficulty with speaking and swallowing grows severe, and patients are ultimately bedridden and demented.

At the time of death, pathologic examination of the brain shows gross atrophy in the caudate and putamen, with lesser change in the pallidum and minor changes in the neocortex (Fig. 5-9). There is glial cell reaction in the striatum, with loss of intrinsic nerve cells, especially stellate cells. Staining of tissue for NADPH-diaphorase shows that a population of aspinous small cells are selectively preserved. Passing fibers (axons) and terminals of extrinsic afferents are preserved throughout, including those from the cortex and substantia nigra. Biochemical studies of postmortem brain show changes in a variety of relevant neurotransmitter systems. Unlike Parkinson's disease, Huntington's disease is not a disorder of a single cell class.

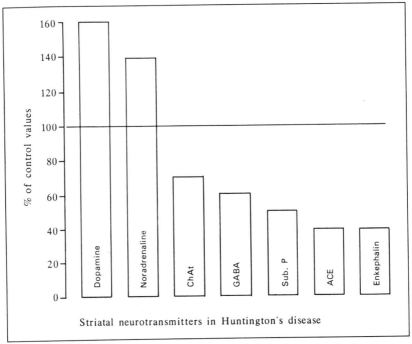

FIGURE 5-10. Neurotransmitter content of the striatum (caudate and puta-men) in Huntington's disease. Data come from biochemical studies of post-mortem brain. ChAt = choline acetyltransferase, a marker for cholinergic neurons; GABA = γ-aminobutyric acid; Sub. P = substance P; ACE = angiotensin converting enzyme. (Adapted from C.D. Marsden, Basal gan-glia disease. *Lancet* 2 : 1144, 1982, with permission.)

Acetylcholine, γ-aminobutyric acid (GABA), substance P, and enkeph-alin are all decreased in tissue (Fig. 5-10). These transmitters are mark-ers of intrinsic and projection neurons. Dopamine concentration in the striatum is *increased*, a phenomenon related to loss of bulk. The preservation of afferents from the substantia nigra results in a relative increase in dopamine as other tissue is lost. Somatostatin and neu-ropeptide Y are likewise increased; these peptides are localized in some of the aspinous stellate cells that are spared.

Alteration of Motor Control in Huntington's Disease

The early abnormality of motor control in Huntington's disease is chorea: irregular, extraneous involuntary movements. An attractive hypothesis relates the movements to the loss of small cells and relative excess of dopaminergic influence in the striatum. The disturbance of function in the striatal loop is the opposite of that in Parkinson's disease. Abnormal regulation of striatopallidal activity results in excess movement. There is failure to suppress extraneous motor routines, which are run together with normal movement. There is lack of persistence at ongoing motor tasks. As predicted, levodopa aggravates chorea in Huntington's disease. Drugs that reduce dopamine synaptic function, such as reserpine, chlorpromazine, and haloperidol, *decrease* choreic movements.

Late in the illness, loss of striatal neurons limits motor function in a more basic way. Striatopallidal processing decreases when cell loss is great. Rigidity and dystonia are more pronounced, and the chorea is less. Abnormal involuntary movements are not the limiting feature in advanced Huntington's disease. Patients are more disabled by mental impairment.

The Cause of Cell Death in Huntington's Disease

Huntington's disease is a dominantly inherited disorder, in which cell loss begins sometime during adult life. Patients are born with a normal nervous system. Once the disease process begins, neuronal loss is selective, even in regions most severely affected. In the caudate, for example, a subset of NADPH-diaphorase–positive stellate cells is spared. An attractive theory relates selective cell loss in Huntington's disease to neurotoxic properties of excitatory amino acids and their analogs.

Glutamate is ubiquitous in the forebrain. Excitatory pathways from the cortex to the striatum utilize glutamate as the principal neurotransmitter. Glutamate receptors are widely distributed in caudate and putamen. The three principal types of glutamate receptor are characterized by their preferred agonist: kianate, quisqualate, or N-methyl-*d*-aspartate (NMDA, Fig. 5-11). Though glutamate is normally present in nervous tissues, Olney and others have demonstrated that excess exposure to glutamate can be toxic to neurons. At the NMDA receptor, glutamate opens channels for sodium and calcium entrance into the nerve cell. Unopposed, chronic exposure results in swelling and death of postsynaptic neurons. The osmotic swelling is mediated by entry of sodium (and chloride) into the cell. The delayed cell death appears to be mediated by calcium, as it can be prevented in tissue culture by removing calcium from the medium. Fortunately, mechanisms exist in nervous tissue for handling glutamate, principally by uptake into glial cells and nerve terminals. Injury to adult nervous tissues from excess synaptic release of glutamate does not occur under normal physiologic conditions.

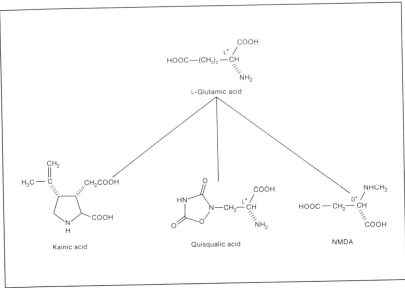

FIGURE 5-11. Preferred agonists for the three major categories of excitatory amino acid (glutamate) receptor.

Kianic acid and quinolinic acid have been studied for their excitant toxin properties. Quinolinic acid is an analog of glutamate, which acts at the NMDA-type glutamate receptor. It binds the receptor with high affinity and opens ion channels. Its excitant effect is ultimately toxic to the postsynaptic nerve cell. It is present in nervous tissues in small quantity as a tryptophan metabolite, but at normal concentrations is not toxic to nervous structures. Beal and Martin suggest one hypothesis for the selective neuronal injury observed in Huntington's disease. They propose that patients may be unable to handle quinolinic acid normally. Nervous tissues of young animals are less vulnerable, but the toxin may accumulate in the adult to cause progressive loss of neurons. Those cells which contain the diaphorase enzyme may be able to metabolize quinolinic acid and avoid injury. Injection of quinolinic acid into the striatum causes an injury pattern in intrinsic neurons which mimics the cellular pathology of Huntington's disease.

The nitrile family of centrally acting neurotoxins may also have an excitotoxin mechanism. Beta-N-oxalylamino-l-alanine (BOAA) is found in the chickling pea, *Lathyrus sativus*. Long-term dietary exposure causes a chronically progressive spastic paraparesis, a syndrome known as *neurolathyrism*. A related toxin has been linked to a form of motor neuron disease found among the Chamorro population of Guam. Beta-N-methylamino-l-alanine (BMAA) is found in the seed of the cycad plant, an inexpensive and ubiquitous source of protein used by the natives to make flour tortillas. Recent animal studies by Spenser et al. indicate that these toxins, which are amino acid analogs, act at the excitatory amino acid (glutamate) receptor. Receptor blocking drugs may provide an approach to intervention in these diseases, though avoidance of the toxic substance would provide more direct benefits.

TARDIVE DYSKINESIA

Tardive dyskinesia is a common movement disorder problem, which is wholly iatrogenic (induced inadvertently by the treatment of a physician). The phenothiazine antipsychotic drugs were introduced into clinical practice in the 1950s. This family of drugs has powerful effects on thought disorder (delusions, hallucinations) and on behavior in schizophrenic patients. The drugs have revolutionized psychiatric practice, reduced the rate of relapse, and permitted many chronic patients to function in the community. The drugs share the property of antagonism and binding at the postsynaptic dopamine receptor complex. Their antipsychotic potency is directly proportional to their effect on dopamine receptor binding in vitro (Fig. 5-12). The drugs also antagonize dopamine receptors in the motor system. The tendency of these drugs in large dose to make animals stiff and rigid is known as the *neuroleptic* effect. The neuroleptic drugs can induce parkinsonism in human patients, a side effect which diminishes as the drug is cleared.

Ten to forty percent of patients treated with these powerful medications develop involuntary movements. *Tardive dyskinesia* refers to a syndrome of choreic movements in patients on neuroleptic drugs, movements which are late in onset and persist when the medication is withdrawn. More than 6 months' exposure is generally required to produce the disorder; in some patients the effect is irreversible. Movements most often begin in the lips, tongue, and jaw. They may involve the limbs and trunk, and then resemble the chorea of Huntington's disease, though the movements of tardive dyskinesia are more repetitive and stereotyped. Tardive dyskinesia is not a universal occurrence in patients on neuroleptic drugs. Increased risk is associated with some identifiable factors, including age and sex of the patient.

Synaptic Basis of the Movement Disorder

In order to understand the mechanism of the movement disorder, we need to examine events at the receptor level. An animal model exists,

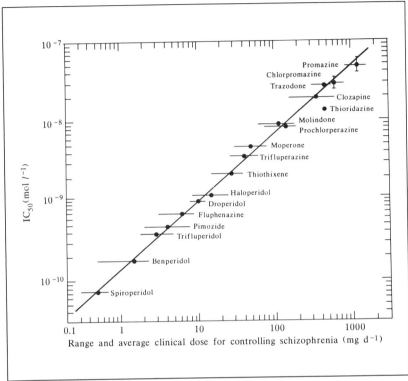

FIGURE 5-12. Potency of dopamine receptor binding (IC_{50}), compared with antipsychotic effect for the commonly used antipsychotic drugs. The IC_{50} is the quantity that reduces the stereospecific binding of ^{3}H-halperidol by 50 percent. (From M. Lipton et al. [eds.], *Psychopharmacology: A Generation of Progress.* New York: Raven Press, 1978, p. 950, with permission.)

created by chronic administration of neuroleptic drugs to animals. In rats so treated, odd stereotyped behaviors such as licking and gnawing can be elicited, particularly after treatment with dopamine agonist drugs. Unlike the human disorder, the effect in animals is universal and is reversible. When the brain is examined, striatal homogenate shows increased binding at the dopamine receptor complex, compared to control animals. A popular hypothesis regards this finding as evidence of postsynaptic supersensitivity to dopamine. Recall what happens at the neuromuscular junction or peripheral autonomic synapse in response to denervation. A proliferation of postsynaptic receptor is observed, with enhanced sensitivity to neurotransmitter (Fig. 5-13). This phenomenon in the peripheral nervous system is known as *denervation supersensitivity.*

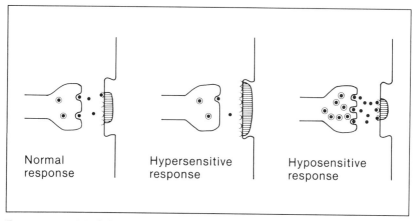

| Normal response | Hypersensitive response | Hyposensitive response |

FIGURE 5-13. Modulation of the synapse: A prolonged change in activity of the presynaptic neuron results in a modification of the synapse, with altered postsynaptic sensitivity to neurotransmitter. This effect is particularly marked after denervation of skeletal muscle or autonomic ganglia, where a proliferation of postsynaptic receptor is observed (denervation supersensitivity).

By analogy, this hypothesis regards tardive dyskinesia as a syndrome of dopaminergic hyperfunction. Chronic neuroleptic exposure produces altered regulation of the postsynaptic receptor, resulting in enhanced sensitivity to endogenous dopamine. As in Huntington's disease, excess dopamine function disturbs motor production in the striatal loop, resulting in excess, involuntary movement. The response of tardive dyskinesia to drug treatment confirms the predictions of the model: drugs that increase dopamine synaptic function make the movements worse. Reserpine, alpha-methyltyrosine, and drugs that decrease dopamine synaptic function reduce the movements. There is a temptation to suppress tardive dyskinesia by restarting or increasing the neuroleptic dose. Unfortunately, this approach aggravates the underlying disorder, and risks more serious adverse drug reactions. Choline and lecithin, substances which enhance CNS synthesis of acetylcholine, have a transient beneficial effect in some individuals with tardive dyskinesia.

TREMOR

Many other involuntary movement disorders are encountered in practice. Dystonia, myoclonus, and tic syndromes are not fully understood, and are outside the scope of this chapter. Tremor is a relatively

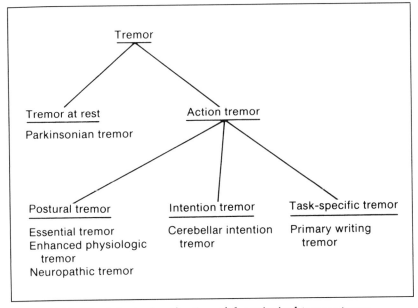

FIGURE 5-14. Physiologic classification of the principal tremor types.

common problem, and the physiology is somewhat better known. A *tremor* is an oscillating involuntary movement across a joint. Tremors are typically classified into tremor with movement (action tremor) and tremor at rest (resting tremor, Fig. 5-14). Tremors occurring on movement are further divided into postural tremor (enhanced physiologic tremor, essential/familial tremor), cerebellar intention tremor, and tremor restricted to a particular task, such as writing tremor.

Tremor at Rest

Resting tremor is characteristic of Parkinson's disease. It occurs at 3 to 7 cps, and is most prominent in the distal upper extremities ("pill-rolling tremor"). It diminishes in intensity with limb use, which distinguishes it from the group of action tremors. An alternating pattern of electromyographic (EMG) activity is recorded in agonist and antagonist muscles. The oscillation is generated centrally in Parkinson's disease, most likely related to a disorder of thalamocortical activity. Dopamine replacement therapy reduces parkinsonian tremor. Lesions in the ventrolateral thalamic nucleus eliminate tremor on the contralateral side. Procedures such as dorsal rhizotomy, which interrupt the segmental stretch reflex, do not affect the tremor.

Tremor with Movement

A small amount of tremor is present in each of us, tremor that can be brought out by fatigue, stress, thyroid hormone, or stimulants. This physiologic tremor becomes symptomatic in some patients. It is an *action tremor*, 8 to 12 cps. Studies suggest that enhanced physiologic tremor is related to overtuning and oscillation in the segmental stretch reflex. A burst of muscle contraction excites the spindle afferents. After a brief delay, reflex firing occurs in the motor unit. In response to muscle action, the spindle afferents are again fired. The activity in the segmental motor pool becomes periodic and synchronized. β-Adrenergic receptor blockers decrease this tremor, acting peripherally on the skeletal muscle. Use (abuse) of these drugs has become a common practice among performing artists.

Essential (familial) tremor is somewhat slower (5–10 cps) and greater in amplitude. It may involve the head or voice. Many patients discover for themselves the remarkable suppressant effect of alcohol on essential tremor. A central mechanism has been proposed, because peripheral injection of β-blockers (or alcohol) does not decrease tremor in a limb. The anatomic substrate for the tremor within the CNS has not been defined.

Cerebellar intention tremor has a different quality. It is a slower, side-to-side oscillation that occurs when a voluntary movement is produced. The tremor amplitude increases as the goal is approached, in a manner most suggestive of a defective servomechanism. Cerebellar tremor is rarely seen in isolation, and almost always as part of a cerebellar syndrome.

CEREBELLAR INFLUENCE ON MOTOR CONTROL

We know a great deal about the synaptic architecture of the cerebellum, yet less about how it does its job. The principal cell type of the cerebellar cortex is the Purkinje cell; its output is uniformly inhibitory. Cells in the cerebellar cortex are active in relation to movement. The anatomic organization suggests that the cerebellum is a motor "co-processor." Nonetheless, motor function is possible without it. With ablation of a cerebellar hemisphere (after extensive neurosurgery or stroke), voluntary movement occurs on the involved side, but the performance is flawed. Gordon Holmes described *ataxia:* the syndrome of disordered motor control seen with cerebellar lesions. Features include dysmetria (the mismeasurement of a movement), intention tremor, difficulty executing rapid alternating movements, hypotonia, and a loss of mechanical damping. Gait, speech, and eye movements are commonly involved. His descriptions provide the basis for our working assumption about the cerebellum—that its role is in the coordination of movement.

Diseases of the cerebellum are common. Multiple sclerosis frequently affects cerebellar connections; strokes and tumors are often seen in this part of the nervous system. Cerebellar degenerations are described, which may be familial or sporadic. A number of toxic or metabolic disturbances affect cerebellar performance disproportionally. Alcohol intoxication is the commonest cause of gait ataxia, a bit of neurology appreciated by the police in screening for drunk drivers. Chronic alcoholics sometimes suffer atrophy of the anterior vermis, a part of the cerebellum that helps coordinate walking. Ataxia and incoordination result from lesions anywhere in the cerebellar system: the cerebellum and its afferent or efferent connections. The lesion need not be in the cerebellum proper. Friedreich's ataxia is a progressive disorder in which most of the pathology is spinal, involving the dorsal and ventral spinocerebellar tracts and Clarke's column. A deafferentated cerebellum functions as poorly as a damaged one.

The Midline Zone

It is helpful to regard the cerebellum as a three-component system. The division into midline, intermediate, and lateral zones is derived from the anatomy of the cerebellum and its efferent connections (Fig. 5-15). The output connections of the cerebellum are routed through the deep nuclei: the fastigial nucleus, the interposed nuclei, and the dentate. The midline zone consists of that part of the cerebellum which projects to the fastigial nuclei: the anterior and posterior vermis, and the medial sector of the flocculonodular lobe. Some parts of the flocculus project directly to the vestibular nucleus. The midline zone influences the function of the vestibulospinal and reticulospinal tracts. This is the phylogenetically oldest part of the cerebellum, well developed in all vertebrates. These structures are concerned with postural support, locomotion, and compensation for movements of the head and eyes.

Lesions in this part of the cerebellum of whatever cause result in imbalance, which is particularly severe in the upright posture. Atrophy

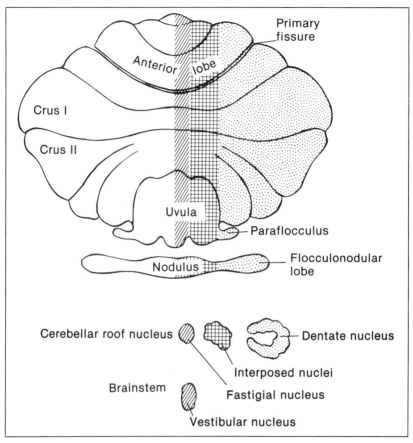

FIGURE 5-15. Zonal organization of the cerebellum: The cerebellum is divided into three sagittal zones, according to the deep nuclei through which it projects (*below*). The lateral zone projects to the lateral, or dentate nucleus. The intermediate zone projects to the interposed nuclei, the globose and emboliform. The midline zone projects to the fastigial nucleus. Parts of the flocculonodular lobe project directly to the vestibular nucleus in the brainstem. (Adapted from A. Brodal. *Neurological Anatomy* [3rd ed.]. New York: Oxford University Press, 1979, p. 299, with permission.)

of the anterior vermis results in gait ataxia and titubation (side-to-side oscillation) of the trunk. Rotated or tilted postures of the head can be observed with lesions in the midline zone. This part of the cerebellum is involved in tuning the vestibulo-ocular reflex. An "error signal" here results in *nystagmus*, a slow drift and rapid refixation in conjugate gaze.

The Intermediate Zone

The intermediate zone consists of the paravermian region, and that part of the lateral hemisphere on either side which projects to the interposed nuclei. These structures have developed markedly in higher animals, especially predators. Afferents to this part of the cerebellum include segments of the dorsal and ventral spinocerebellar tracts. Efferent projections influence the rubrospinal system.

These structures monitor afferents from the muscle spindle and Golgi tendon organs. They regulates tone, and provide feedback control over movement in progress. Some movements are done slowly and carefully, with sensory-motor control and constant refinement. This pattern of closed-loop motor control contrasts with the rapid execution of preprogrammed motor routines described above. The closed-loop mode is particularly suited to exploration and motor learning. There is considerable evidence to suggest that the intermediate zone functions as a *comparator*. It receives information from the mossy fiber pathways on plans for intended movement *and* spinal afferents reporting on movement in progress. Corrections are relayed back to the red nucleus and thalamus to modify ongoing performance.

The cerebellum adjusts tone, and thereby helps damp oscillations. In its absence, tremor is observed, and the extended limb may rebound abnormally after a perturbation.

The Lateral Zone (Neocerebellum)

The lateral zone includes the lateral cerebellar hemispheres, that region which projects to the dentate nucleus. This component system is particularly developed in primates, animals with dexterity and opposable digits. Cells in the dentate nucleus are active 100 msec before voluntary movement, 40 msec prior to the upper motor neuron. This part of the cerebellum, together with the basal ganglia, helps in the planning and production of skilled movements. Experts believe it contributes information on muscle burst duration and timing. Skilled hand movements are possible without cerebellar input, but at some sacrifice in dexterity. The fine tuning of motor performance, the precise coordinated action of different muscle groups, relies on this structure. Dysmetria and past pointing are observed with lateralized lesions of the cerebellar hemisphere, as well as a general loss in synergy of muscle action (decomposition of movement). Rapid alternating movements or fine repetitive movements in particular are poorly executed.

BIBLIOGRAPHY

Baldessarini, R.J., and Tarsy, D. Dopamine and the pathophysiology of dyskinesias induced by antipsychotic drugs, *Annu. Rev. Neurosci.* 3 : 23–41, 1980.

Eccles, J. The Control of Movement by the Brain. In J. Eccles (ed.), *The Understanding of the Brain.* New York: McGraw-Hill, 1977. Pp. 106–144.

Holmes, G. The cerebellum of man. *Brain* 62 : 1–30, 1939.

Lawrence, D.G., and Kuypers, H. The functional organization of the motor system in the monkey. *Brain* 91 : 1–36, 1968.

Marsden, C.D., and Parkes, J.D. Success and problems of long-term levodopa therapy in Parkinson's disease. *Lancet* 1 : 345–349, 1977.

Martin, J.B. Huntington's disease: New approaches to an old problem. *Neurology* 34 : 1059–1071, 1984.

Penny, J.B., and Young, A.B. Speculations on the functional anatomy of basal ganglia disorders. *Annu. Rev. Neurosci.* 6 : 73–94, 1983.

Snyder, S.H., and D'Amato, R.J. MPTP: A neurotoxin relevant to the pathophysiology of Parkinson's disease, *Neurology* 36 : 250–258, 1986.

Ungerstedt, U. Functional Dynamics of Central Monoamine Pathways. In F.O. Schmidt and F.G. Worden (eds.), *The Neurosciences: Third Study Program*, Cambridge, Mass.: MIT Press, 1974. Pp. 979–989.

PART III

Cerebral Cortex: Consciousness, Mental State, and Behavior

CHAPTER 6

Consciousness and Its Disorders

Consciousness is a being such that, in its being, its being is constantly in question, insofar as its being implies a being other than itself.
Jean-Paul Sartre

Almost every psychologist or philosopher has pondered the problem of consciousness. William James envisioned consciousness as a dynamic entity, as a stream of mental process. Freud concerned himself largely with events outside of conscious awareness. Consciousness is a state of mind, intuitively understood, but difficult to characterize. Its essence is awareness, and the capacity for self-reflection. Eccles and Popper regard consciousness as an emergent property of higher nervous systems. An emergent property is only meaningful when a given level of organizational complexity is attained. We cannot regard consciousness as having a molecular basis, nor as an aspect of cell or tissue culture. We can speak of the collective consciousness of a crowd or even a nation.

At what level does consciousness emerge? The ability to monitor its processes (i.e., to reflect on itself) is a property of a more complex nervous system. Domestic animals are undoubtedly capable of sufficient presence of mind to do this. It is difficult to say at what point in evolution mental function became adequately complex to support conscious thought. Is a frog conscious, or an ant? The human neonate is unquestionably a conscious being, although asleep most of the time. Most experts believe that consciousness begins at birth, though some question whether the human fetus in the third trimester has some nascent consciousness. This question is especially difficult to resolve, given the complex range of ethical and legal issues surrounding the status of the fetus. We do not generally regard the most powerful digital computer as having a consciousness, though its competence may be greater than the infant human.

For medical purposes, consciousness is best defined through the study of its absence. The properties of the unconscious state reveal a great deal about the normal operations of the nervous system. Plum and Posner, in their monograph on stupor and coma, define consciousness as "the state of awareness of the self and the environment." They describe two components of the conscious state: *Content*

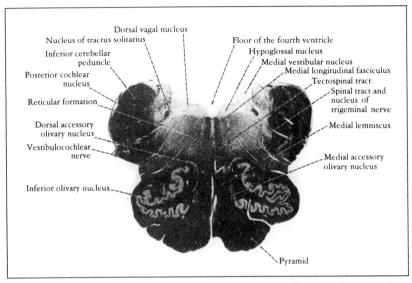

FIGURE 6-1. Myelin-stained section through the medulla at the level of the inferior olive. Reticular formation is in the tegmentum, and has a reticulated, or ground-glass appearance in this preparation. (From R. Snell, *Clinical Neuroanatomy for Medical Students* [2nd ed.]. Boston: Little, Brown, 1987, p. 190, with permission.)

of consciousness is the sum of mental function, the collection of thoughts entertained by the nervous system at a given point in time. *Arousal* is the behavioral appearance of wakefulness. Either can fail independently of the other. A patient may appear awake, yet have nothing on his mind. Another patient, after an overdose of sedatives, can process information briefly when roused, but may be unable to stay awake for more than a few moments.

ANATOMIC SUBSTRATE FOR CONSCIOUSNESS

Like other nervous system functions, consciousness can be localized. The content of consciousness reflects the activity of the cerebral cortex. The cortex is the structure that supports conscious awareness. Arousal, on the other hand, is mediated by phylogenetically older structures in the brainstem core. The arousal system resides in the brainstem reticular formation.

The Reticular Formation

The reticular formation was described by nineteenth century neuroanatomists, who observed that parts of the brainstem had a reticulate

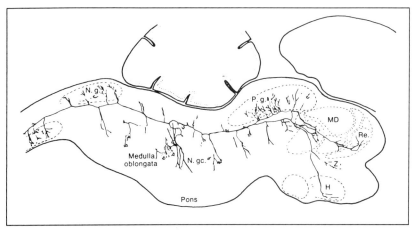

FIGURE 6-2. Drawing of a sagittal section from the brainstem of a 2-day-old rat, prepared with the Golgi stain. A single large cell in the magnocellular nucleus is shown. It emits an axon which bifurcates into an ascending and descending branch. The latter gives off collaterals to the nucleus gracilis (N. g.), and to the ventral horn of the spinal cord. The ascending branch gives off collaterals to the periaqueductal gray (P.g.); it then appears to supply several thalamic nuclei, the hypothalamus (H), and the zona incerta (Z). N. gc. = nucleus gigantocellularis; MD = medial dorsal nucleus of the thalamus; Re. = reticular thalamic nucleus. (From M. Scheibel and A. Scheibel. Structural Substrates for Integrative Patterns in the Brain Stem Reticular Core. In H.H. Jasper et al. [eds.], *Reticular Formation of the Brain. Henry Ford Hospital International Symposium.* Boston: Little, Brown, 1958, pp. 31–46, with permission.)

appearance on myelin-stained sections (Fig. 6-1). These areas are the parts left over after cranial nerve nuclei, cerebellar connections, and long tracts are identified. Within this region is a network of diffusely projecting neurons. Several nuclear groups have been identified, containing some of the largest cells in the nervous system. There is a general correlation between neuronal size and the volume of axon process the cell needs to maintain. The colossal neurons of the nucleus gigantocellularis (Fig. 6-2) project up into the basal forebrain and thalamus, and down into the spinal cord. Projections of reticular neurons extend into every part of the neuraxis. The reticular formation is not somatotopically organized in any recognizable way. Rather its connections span different functional systems. The pain pathway, the autonomic nervous system, and the limbic system are sources of afferents to the reticular formation.

Consider the functional implications of such a system. With its remote ramifications, the reticular formation is thought to generate a baseline state for the nervous system. Nauta suggests that the reticular formation produces a "posture" for central nervous system (CNS) response. It is a center for control over the day-to-day function of the viscera, and control over aspects of postural support and locomotion. It activates higher centers, contributing to the alerting response, vigilance, and arousal from sleep. Sleep itself depends on structures within the reticular formation.

Reticular Activating System

The reticular activating system was described by physiologists in the 1940s and 1950s. Within the reticular formation is that part of the brainstem which mediates the alerting response. Structures between the rostral pons and caudal diencephalon are necessary for arousal. Lesions of the upper brainstem tegmentum in animals result in a state of persistent unresponsiveness. The animals never regain consciousness. Stimulation of this region in a sleeping animal produces arousal. In a waking animal, stimulation evokes behavioral and electroencephalographic (EEG) manifestations of the alerting response. In sum, the reticular activating system appears to be the substrate for arousal.

The tegmentum of the upper pons and midbrain also serves other vital functions. Conjugate eye movements are generated here. The pupillary light reflex is mediated by structures in the pretectal area of the midbrain. The corneal reflex (fifth and seventh cranial nerves) passes through the pons. These primitive responses serve as markers for the structural integrity of the brainstem core. Neurologic injury here results in abnormality of one or more of these basic functions.

Cerebral Cortex and Consciousness

The cortical mantle of the hemispheres is the organ of conscious thought. Higher processing, which gives content to the waking state, occurs when the cortex is activated. The cortex is a connection machine, specialized for associative thought. Its architecture and detailed function are reviewed in Chapter 8.

The cerebral cortex is reliant on subcortical structures for much of its afferent information. Thalamic nuclei project to sensory and motor cortical structures, as reviewed in Chapters 4 and 5. Ninety to ninety-five percent of the thalamus projects in this manner to specific cortical fields. The rest of the thalamus is comprised of intralaminar and reticular thalamic nuclei. These regions, within the interstices, project more diffusely. Through these structures, the reticular activating system promotes cortical processing.

The effect can be observed in surface recordings of cortical activity, done with scalp electrodes (EEG). The basis for the EEG waveform is described in Chapter 7. For the present, the EEG can be regarded as a recording of cerebral activity, averaged over millions of individual

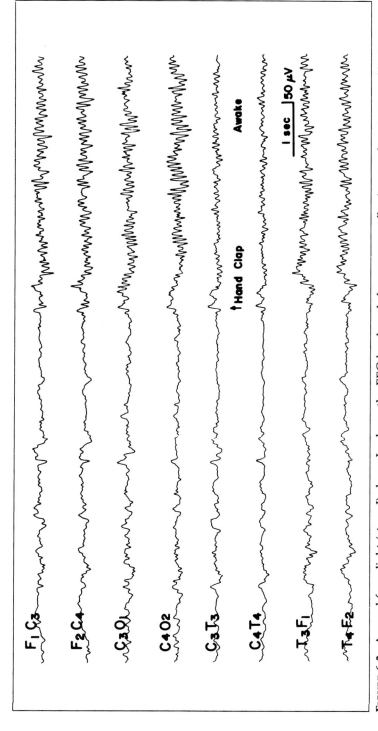

FIGURE 6-3. Arousal from light (stage I) sleep. In sleep, the EEG has broad slow waves, reflecting synchronization of brain electrical activity. After a loud noise (*arrow*), there is return of the waking pattern. (From D. Klass and D. Daly, *Current Practice of Clinical EEG*. New York: Raven Press, 1979, p. 125, with permission.)

cortical neurons. When we relax, sit back, and smell the roses, thalamic driving tends to synchronize the EEG. This produces intrinsic rhythms, or "waves" of brain electrical activity. The effect is even more dramatic when we drift off into sleep. Stimulating the reticular activating system desynchronizes EEG activity, a correlate of the alerting response (Fig. 6-3).

Brainstem Monoamine Pathways

Since the first descriptions of the reticular activating system, there has been a methodologic revolution in the neurosciences. It is now possible to map specific neurotransmitter pathways. This revolution began with the discovery by Falck and Hillarp in the late 1960s of catecholamine histofluorescence. Monoamine-containing nerve cells and their processes can be made to exhibit fluorescence when exposed to formaldehyde vapor. Using histochemical techniques, it has been possible to identify and map the discrete monoamine pathways within the CNS.

Many of the neurons within the reticular formation are cholinergic; like the motor neuron, they rely on acetylcholine as their neurotransmitter. Within the anatomic boundaries of the brainstem reticular formation, however, are several nuclear groups which contain monoamines. These are the site of origin of extensive projection systems for dopamine, norepinephrine, and serotonin.

The substantia nigra and the adjacent ventral tegmental area are the root of the forebrain dopamine system. The substantia nigra projects to the caudate and putamen, as reviewed in Chapter 5, while the adjacent ventral tegmental area projects to the nucleus accumbens, olfactory tubercle, and mesial frontal lobe. The locus ceruleus, a small pigmented nuclear group in the pontine tegmentum, projects diffusely. It is the site of origin for virtually all the norepinephrine innervation of the forebrain and spinal cord (Fig. 6-4). The various nuclei of the median raphe contain serotonin projections, which are also widely distributed (Fig. 6-5).

Considering the global functions of the reticular formation, what specific role might we assign to these amine systems? The dopamine pathways are involved in the initiation and maintenance of movement. The mesocortical-mesolimbic dopamine system (ventral tegmental area) is thought to be important for motivation. The functions of the locus ceruleus pathway have been extensively examined. Recent studies have suggested a role in the modulation of attention. The norepinepherine system may have something to do with global orientation and vigilance. This pathway may function in parallel with the diffuse thalamocortical projection system in the alerting response. A substantial literature suggests a role for the locus coeruleus in the

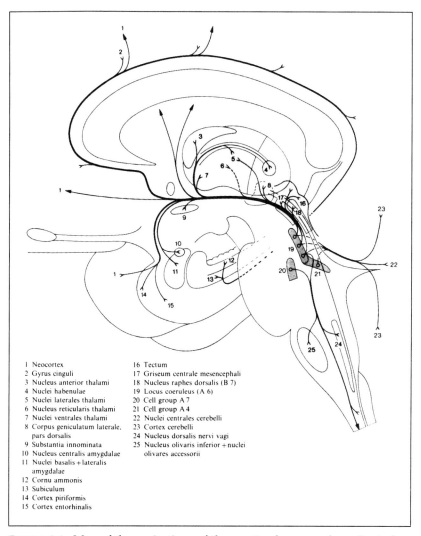

1 Neocortex
2 Gyrus cinguli
3 Nucleus anterior thalami
4 Nuclei habenulae
5 Nuclei laterales thalami
6 Nuclei reticularis thalami
7 Nuclei ventrales thalami
8 Corpus geniculatum laterale, pars dorsalis
9 Substantia innominata
10 Nucleus centralis amygdalae
11 Nuclei basalis + lateralis amygdalae
12 Cornu ammonis
13 Subiculum
14 Cortex piriformis
15 Cortex entorhinalis
16 Tectum
17 Griseum centrale mesencephali
18 Nucleus raphes dorsalis (B 7)
19 Locus coeruleus (A 6)
20 Cell group A 7
21 Cell group A 4
22 Nuclei centrales cerebelli
23 Cortex cerebelli
24 Nucleus dorsalis nervi vagi
25 Nucleus olivaris inferior + nuclei olivares accessorii

FIGURE 6-4. Map of the projections of the pontine locus ceruleus. Rostral projections travel along the medial forebrain bundle through the hypothalamus and septal area. (From R. Nieuwenhuys, J. Voogd, and C. van Huijzen, *The Human Central Nervous System* [2nd ed.]. New York: Springer-Verlag, 1981, p. 228, with permission.)

cyclic generation of sleep states. The projections of the raphe nuclei, the serotonin pathways, are least understood. Some role has been suggested with regard to pain control, sleep, and thermoregulation. (The apparent role of serotonin and norepinephrine systems in the modulation of affect and behavior is not well understood. Most antidepressant drugs effect the synaptic action of the monoamines in some way.)

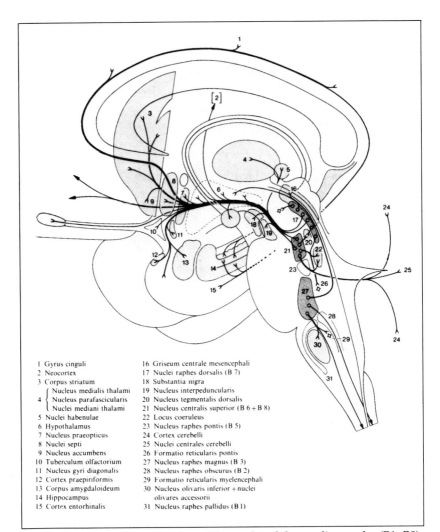

FIGURE 6-5. The serotonin system. The nuclei of the median raphe (B1–B8) are found in man along the brainstem tegmentum, within the boundaries of the reticular formation. (From R. Nieuwenhuys, J. Voogd, and C. van Huijzen, *The Human Central Nervous System* [2nd ed.]. New York: Springer-Verlag, 1981, p. 230, with permission.)

COMA

Coma is defined as the pathologic absence of consciousness. The patient cannot be roused enough to interact. Failure of arousal mechanisms can be observed in degrees. *Lethargy* is a state in which the patient appears asleep, but can be aroused by the examiner's voice.

Stupor is a deeper state, in which arousal requires uncomfortable tactile stimulation, and does not persist for more than a few moments. *Deep coma* is an unconscious state from which the patient can no longer be aroused by any combination of stimuli. For practical purposes, a description of the patient's state in plain language is often the best. (e.g., "Patient moans, and opens his eyes briefly when his name is called." "Irregular breathing, postures to sternal rub.") Coma suggests serious illness, and is a true medical emergency.

The physiology of coma can be understood in terms of the substrate for the conscious state detailed above. Three mechanisms are described: (1) Patients may suffer a depression of cortical function, a failure of cerebral processing. (2) Patients may lack brainstem arousal systems. (3) Some patients become unconscious when the functions of the reticular system are disturbed by an expanding mass.

Coma Due to Diffuse Cerebral Cortical Failure

Depression of function in both cerebral hemispheres results in loss of consciousness. Some degree of sleepiness may be seen with a large stroke confined to one hemisphere, but the presence of stupor or coma implies failure of a substantial mass of cerebral cortex on both sides. Brainstem functions of the reticular system are preserved, but activation fails at the cortical level. This type of failure is sometimes seen with extensive structural damage. Bilateral carotid stroke, meningitis, or encephalitis can cause coma through this mechanism. More commonly, the disturbance is related to toxins or metabolic failure.

Disturbance of cerebral function due to drug effect or metabolic disorder is called toxic or metabolic *encephalopathy*. In mild degree, metabolic encephalopathy results in confusion (see Delirium, below). In severe degree, loss of consciousness can occur. The commonest cause of coma, diffuse encephalopathy, is identified in roughly 60 percent of patients. Half of these cases are due to drug toxicity. Overdosage with narcotics, sedative-hypnotics, or more exotic contemporary drugs is a common emergency room problem. This phenomenon bridges socioeconomic class differences although narcotic overdose is somewhat more prevalent among the urban poor.

The various causes of metabolic brain failure are reviewed in Chapter 10. Some form of oxygen or substrate deprivation is the most common. Cerebral injury due to hypotension or cardiac arrest is the most frequent cause of coma *inside* the hospital. Any disorder adversely affecting the neuron's metabolic milieu can cause encephalopathy. This category includes extreme hypothermia, and extreme degrees of electrolyte disorder (hypercalcemia, hyponatremia, diabetic ketoacidosis, hyperosmolar state).

Patients with hepatic failure have a particular variety of metabolic coma. They exhibit hypersomnolence with asterixis (150-msec lapse in tonic innervation of muscle), hyperventilation, and large-amplitude slow waves on the EEG. The disorder is correlated with hepatocellular dysfunction, impaired handling of amino acids, and an inability to clear ammonia. It is particularly common in patients with portacaval shunting of venous blood. The cause of hepatic coma is not fully understood. One hypothesis suggests that ammonia itself, or perhaps some related compound, acts as a neurotoxin. A more likely explanation focuses on the disorder of cerebral energy metabolism which results from the amination of Krebs cycle metabolites. Perhaps the most intriguing hypothesis considers the impact of the metabolic disorder on neurotransmitters. Glutamate and aspartate are excitatory transmitters in the cerebral cortex, and γ-aminobutyric acid (GABA) is the principal inhibitory transmitter. As the metabolic pool of glutamate is depleted, the neurotransmitter pool may become deficient.

Primary Brainstem Failure

Failure of arousal mechanisms due to brainstem disease is the cause of coma in roughly 15 percent of patients. The syndrome results from destruction of brainstem tissue, and compromise of the reticular activating system. This outcome can be observed after basilar artery stroke, pontine hemorrhage, or destruction of the brainstem from an adjacent posterior fossa tumor.

This state is characterized by the loss of ocular reflexes which reside in the upper brainstem tegmentum. In particular, failure of the pupillary light reflex, and the corneal, oculocephalic, and/or vestibulocular reflexes points to destruction of the vital core of the upper brainstem. (This inference is not reliable in the presence of barbiturates or other sedative drugs, which may depress brainstem function.)

Compression of the Reticulothalamic System from an Expanding Mass

Expansion of a mass in the cerebral hemispheres can result in displacement of vital structures and failure of arousal. This is the cause of coma in 20 percent of patients. The intracranial compartment has restricted capacity to accommodate a space-occupying lesion. When a mass in the hemispheres grows to occupy 30 to 60 cc, something has to "give" and intracranial structures shift. Studies from the neurological intensive care unit (ICU) indicate that depression of consciousness is correlated with lateral displacement of diencephalic structures. Horizontal shift at the level of the pineal of 3 to 5 mm is regularly associated with drowsiness, 6 to 8 mm with stupor, and above 8 mm with coma.

With progression, the mass can displace the uncus of the temporal lobe, which herniates through the tentorium against the midbrain. Brainstem compression is a common mode of exodus for patients with subdural hematoma, intracerebral hemorrhage, or brain tumor. The mechanics that underlie the uncal syndrome are reviewed in Chapter 9. A characteristic clinical picture is observed. The third cranial nerve is at risk, sandwiched between the uncus and the brainstem (Fig. 6-6). Trouble is first evident when the ipsilateral pupil becomes dilated and sluggishly reactive to light (early third cranial nerve stage). There is usually some degree of lethargy associated. As the displacement increases, lethargy turns to stupor, and the third cranial nerve failure becomes complete (late third cranial nerve stage). This is usually the limit of reversibility. Sometimes the contralateral cerebral peduncle is compressed against the tentorium on the opposite side (Kernohan's notch), producing an ipsilateral hemiparesis. As events progress, both pupils become fixed to light, the respiratory pattern is altered, and deep coma is attained as the reticular functions fail. In this midbrain stage, decerebrate rigidity is observed. All motor tracts above the vestibular nuclei are disconnected, and the patient responds to stimuli with extensor posturing (see Chapt. 5).

In the evaluation of the comatose patient, the three patterns of failure can be distinguished at the bedside, based on a 5-minute clinical assessment. In this context, the physical examination is more useful than brain imaging technology (such as computed tomography) in making a preliminary diagnosis and management plan. A large series of consecutive coma cases from the emergency service of New York Hospital is listed in Table 6-1. Diffuse cerebral cortical disorders were the predominant category (65%), with drug overdose being the single most common diagnosis.

Other Altered States Simulating Coma

Not every unresponsive patient is unconscious. With *akinetic mutism*, the patient appears behaviorally awake, but does not interact with his environment. The patient's eyes are open and follow the examiner, and the patient appears to attend. There is no speech and no motor output. The patient is mentally "all dressed up with nowhere to go."

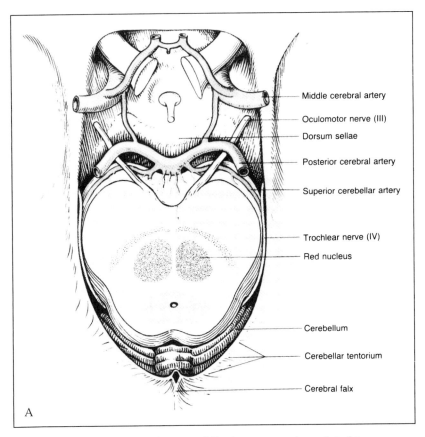

Middle cerebral artery

Oculomotor nerve (III)

Dorsum sellae

Posterior cerebral artery

Superior cerebellar artery

Trochlear nerve (IV)

Red nucleus

Cerebellum

Cerebellar tentorium

Cerebral falx

A

FIGURE 6-6. The uncal syndrome: midbrain compression related to an expanding mass. A. Contents of the tentorial opening (*left*) are viewed from above. The third cranial nerve is at risk, as it is trapped between the posterior cerebral and superior cerebellar artery, along the path of the advancing temporal lobe (uncus). B. Contents of the tentorium are viewed from below, looking up at the forebrain. Extrusion of the uncus (*left*) results in brainstem compression, with secondary hemorrhage and mashing of the contralateral cerebral peduncle. (Reprinted by permission from Duus, P: *Topical Diagnosis in Neurology.* Thieme Medical Publishers, New York, 1983.)

This is a motivation failure, such that the conscious patient does not effect any behavior. Small lesions in the basal forebrain or orbital frontal region can produce this state. The medial forebrain bundle, particularly the mesocortical dopamine pathway, may be important in the activation failure observed. In one patient described by Ross, a man with involvement of orbital frontal structures by a suprasellar tumor, the behavioral deficit was reversed with a dopamine agonist drug. Lesions in the medial dorsal thalamus have also been described with akinetic mutism.

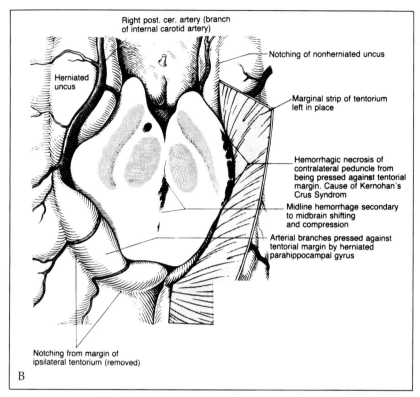

Right post. cer. artery (branch of internal carotid artery)

Notching of nonherniated uncus

Herniated uncus

Marginal strip of tentorium left in place

Hemorrhagic necrosis of contralateral peduncle from being pressed against tentorial margin. Cause of Kernohan's Crus Syndrom

Midline hemorrhage secondary to midbrain shifting and compression

Arterial branches pressed against tentorial margin by herniated parahippocampal gyrus

Notching from margin of ipsilateral tentorium (removed)

B

FIGURE 6-6 (Continued).

After infarction of the basis pontis, patients may be left awake and conscious, but paralyzed. This is known as the *locked-in syndrome*. The patient has no speech output, and no motor activity, with the usual exception of eye movements. Some patients can be trained to communicate using their directed gaze or eye blinks. This syndrome is often compared with the vivid descriptions of the internment of the Count of Monte Cristo. Because the upper brainstem tegmentum is spared, the reticular system and consciousness mechanisms are preserved.

Unconsciousness After Head Injury (Concussion)

Head injury is an important public health problem. Each year there are millions of emergency room visits, and a half million hospitalizations for head injury. Most of these are accidental injuries related to motor vehicles.

Experts on consciousness mechanisms regard the transient failure that occurs with head injury as an enigma. As a clinical phenomenon,

TABLE 6-1. Cause of Stupor or Coma in
500 Patients Seen at New York Hospital*

I. Supratentorial lesions   101
   A. Rhinencephalic and subcortical destructive lesions   2
      1. Thalamic infarcts   2
   B. Supratentorial mass lesions   99
      1. Hemorrhage   76
         a. Intracerebral   44
            (1) Hypertensive   36
            (2) Vascular anomaly   5
            (3) Other   3
         b. Epidural   4
         c. Subdural   26
         d. Pituitary apoplexy   2
      2. Infarction   9
         a. Arterial occlusions   7
            (1) Thrombotic   5
            (2) Embolic   2
         b. Venous occlusions   2
      3. Tumors   7
         a. Primary   2
         b. Metastatic   5
      4. Abscess   6
         a. Intracerebral   5
         b. Subdural   1
      5. Closed head injury   1
II. Subtentorial lesions   65
   A. Compressive lesions   12
      1. Cerebellar hemorrhage   5
      2. Posterior fossa subdural or extradural hemorrhage   1
      3. Cerebellar infarct   2
      4. Cerebellar tumor   3
      5. Cerebellar abscess   1
      6. Basilar aneurysm   0
   B. Destructive or ischemic lesions   53
      1. Pontine hemorrhage   11
      2. Brainstem infarct   40
      3. Basilar migraine   1
      4. Brainstem demyelination   1
III. Diffuse and/or metabolic brain dysfunction   326
   A. Diffuse intrinsic disorders of brain   38
      1. "Encephalitis" or encephalomyelitis   14
      2. Subarachnoid hemorrhage   13
      3. Concussion and postictal states   9
      4. Primary neuronal disorders   2
   B. Extrinsic and metabolic disorders   288
      1. Anoxia or ischemia   10
      2. Hypoglycemia   16
      3. Nutritional   1
      4. Hepatic encephalopathy   17
      5. Uremia and dialysis   8
      6. Pulmonary disease   3
      7. Endocrine disorders (including diabetes)   12

TABLE 6-1 (Continued).

        8. Remote effects of cancer   0
        9. Drug poisons   149
     10. Ionic and acid-base disorders   12
     11. Temperature regulation   9
     12. Mixed or nonspecific metabolic coma   1
IV. Psychiatric "coma"   8
    A. Conversion reactions   4
    B. Depression   2
    C. Catatonic stupor   2

---

*Represents only patients in whom the initial diagnosis was uncertain and a final diagnosis was established. Thus, obvious diagnoses such as known poisonings and closed head injuries, and never-established diagnoses such as mixed metabolic encephalopathies are underrepresented.

Source: F. Plum and J. Posner, *Diagnosis of Stupor and Coma* (3rd ed.). Philadelphia: Davis, 1980. P. 90.

concussion is fairly well defined. There is brief loss of consciousness, with rapid recovery. There is transient amnesia associated. There is generally no evidence of structural injury. For most, the recovery is quick and uneventful. Some less fortunate individuals are troubled for weeks by persistent headache, dizziness, and inability to concentrate (postconcussive syndrome).

The analogy is often advanced of complex electronics which fail when stressed. The nature of the difficulty is not understood, but failure is thought to occur at the level of the reticular activating system. There is speculation about how mechanical forces might be transformed into electrical impulses. Some experts postulate a diffuse release of neurotransmitters. A component of torsional injury seems especially likely to produce loss of consciousness. Rotation of the cerebrum on the brainstem may stress the ascending reticular pathways. Research on woodpeckers, who brace for repeated cranial deceleration, suggests that linear forces are better tolerated than rotational forces. This fact is also well known to the boxer, whose skill is directed at inducing concussion in his opponent.

Some patients remain unconscious hours to days after head injury as a result of structural damage. The Glasgow Coma Scale has provided a useful measure of the severity of injury, and helpful information about the general prognosis in head-injured patients (Table 6-2). A score of 8 or less is associated with a poor prognosis; 50 percent of these patients ultimately fail to regain consciousness.

Nontraumatic Coma: Making a Prognosis

Patients with "medical coma" have a natural history somewhat different from trauma patients. Common examples are patients unconscious

TABLE 6-2. Glasgow Coma Scale for Evaluation of Head Injury

Test	Response	Score
Eye opening	Spontaneous	4
	To speech	3
	To pain	2
	None	1
Best verbal response	Oriented	5
	Confused	4
	Inappropriate	3
	Incomprehensible	2
	None	1
Best motor response (arm)	Obedience to commands	6
	Localization of pain	5
	Withdrawal response to pain	4
	Flexion response to pain	3
	Extension response to pain	2
	None	1

Source: (From G. Teasdale and B. Jennett, Assessment of coma and impaired consciousness; A practical scale. *Lancet* 2 : 81–84, 1974, with permission.)

from hypotension, massive stroke, or cardiac arrest. A more detailed clinical instrument is needed to assess the patients' prognosis. In nontraumatic injuries, the primitive and synaptically simple brainstem systems are most hearty. Brainstem reflexes, particularly those serving ocular movements, are useful markers of the depth and extent of injury.

Using the results of a large, multi-institution collaborative study, it is possible to compare the unconscious patient with hundreds of similar patients. This comparison provides a statistical measure of expected outcome. Predictive data have been defined, based on the patient's neurologic examination at admission to the hospital, at 24 hours, at 3 days, and at 1 week (Fig. 6-7). These data are useful to patients' physicians and family in setting their expectations.

FIGURE 6-7. Estimating prognosis in nontraumatic coma, based on the experience with 500 patients in a collaborative study. Patients may be compared with those surviving various intervals after the onset of coma, based on simple clinical evaluation. Best levels of recovery within 1 year are given for each of the prognostic groups. No Recov = no recovery; Veg State = vegetative state; Sev Disab = severe disability; Motor = motor responses; Ext = extensor; Flex = flexor. (From D.E. Levy, D. Bates, J.J. Caronna, N.E. Cartlidge, R.E. Knill-Jones, R.H. Lapinski, B.H. Singer, D.A. Shaw, and F. Plum. Prognosis in non-traumatic coma. *Ann. Intern. Med.* 94 : 293–301, 1981, with permission.)

155

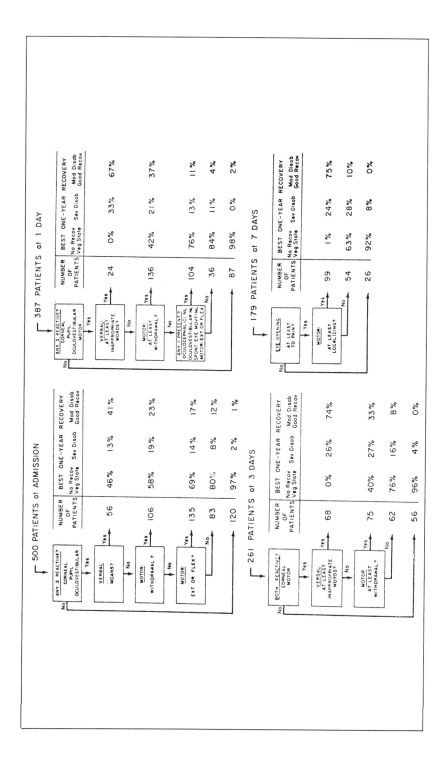

Cerebral Death, Chronic Vegetative State

Death is generally defined as the cessation of heartbeat and respiration. In the modern ICU, it is possible to assist ventilation mechanically, and to support cardiovascular function. As a result, some patients with massive multisystem injury can be kept alive in a condition in which there is little or no nervous system function and no hope for recovery. The law has begun to recognize the importance of defining criteria for *brain death,* to help with decisions about life support and organ donation. The technical requirements of the law vary from state to state. The ultimate goal of these laws is to recognize the irreversible loss of cerebral and brainstem function as the equivalent of death pronounced by traditional means.

Some patients with massive nervous system injury persist in a state of limbo, unable to recover consciousness, yet not meeting the criteria for cerebral death. After 4 to 6 weeks, most such patients will open their eyes, and assume some of the behavioral manifestations of wakefulness. Nonetheless, they are not aware and are unable to interact. This outcome has been termed the *chronic vegetative state.* Law and society have barely begun to wrestle with the implications.

DELIRIUM

Delirium is the commonest disorder of mental state in a general hospital. The essence of the disorder is confusion, the inability to maintain a coherent stream of thought. Confusion results from a failure of attentional mechanisms. The mind is left to wander, and dialogue with the confused patient takes on a certain "scatterbrained" quality. The technical term *delirium* encompasses the acute confusional state, and includes the other disturbances of mental state and behavior that are commonly associated.

The delirious patient has a reduced ability to maintain and fix attention. This core deficit is evident in his speech and behavior. There is also disorganized thinking. Other features that may be present include the following: Some patients exhibit a decreased level of consciousness (lethargy). Patients may show an altered level of activity, either agitation or psychomotor retardation. Hallucinations or perceptual disturbances may be present. A disturbance of the sleep-wake cycle is sometimes observed. Patients may be disoriented. Memory may be impaired. These associated features are not necessary for diagnosis. (The *Diagnostic and Standard Manual of Mental Disorders,* third edition, revised, requires two out of six to sustain a diagnosis.)

Delirium is a diffuse disorder of cerebral function. The mechanisms underlying cerebral activation and attention were reviewed earlier.

TABLE 6-3. Common Causes of Diffuse, Toxic, or Metabolic Encephalopathy

Drug toxicity or withdrawal
  Alcohol
  Narcotic analgesics
  Anticholinergics
  Barbiturates, benzodiazepines, other sedatives
  Psychotropic medications
  Amanita muscaria, peyote, other psychedelic mushrooms
  Cocaine, phencyclidine (PCP), other "recreational drugs"
  Chronic polydrug abuse
Oxygen or substrate deprivation
  Hypoxic/ischemic encephalopathy
  Carbon monoxide poisoning
  Cyanide poisoning
  Hypoglycemia
  Vitamin or cofactor deficiency (B_{12}, thiamine)
Endocrine dysfunction
  Hypothyroidism
  Cushing's syndrome
  Hyperglycemia, diabetic ketoacidosis
  Exogenous steroids (steroid psychosis)
Fluid and electrolyte disorders, acid-base disturbance
  Sodium and water
  Calcium, magnesium
  Acidosis
  Hypercarbia
Failure of other organ systems
  Hepatic failure
  Uremia
  Respiratory failure
Systemic disease
  Hyper-, hypothermia
  Sepsis
Diffuse cerebral injury or dysfunction
  Head trauma
  Postictal state
  Subarachnoid hemorrhage
  Meningitis, encephalitis

A partial list of the conditions which produce delirium is found in Table 6-3. The acute confusional state may be seen with posterior right hemisphere stroke. Otherwise, the list is similar to that for bilateral disorders of cerebral function that produce coma. Delirium may be similar in mechanism to (type I) coma, differing primarily in degree. Most commonly the cause is a toxic or metabolic disturbance, an alteration in function of a structurally intact cerebral cortex. Diseases on this list produce an abnormality at a cellular level, affecting the neuron's metabolic milieu.

The syndrome is important because it is common, usually acute in onset, and generally reversible. Delirium comes on over a period of hours to days, and may fluctuate in intensity. The abnormality of mental state clears over days to a few weeks, once the underlying disorder is successfully treated.

SLEEP

Intuitively, we know the difference between coma and sleep, and we are not alarmed to see someone sleeping (unless he is operating heavy equipment or piloting an airliner). Sleep is an active process, which involves a cyclic pattern of sleep states, dreaming, and considerable movement. The sleeping person can respond to uncomfortable stimuli. Most important, the sleeper is arousable: his or her level of consciousness changes in response to stimulation. We have a basic biologic need for sleep, which varies considerably among individuals. Anywhere from 4 to 10 hours per night may be required. Sleep deprivation experiments show profound changes in physiology and mental performance after just a few days. Recent studies suggest that sleep deprivation and fatigue may influence the performance of house officers working 36-hour shifts on an every-other-night rotation.

Events of the Sleep Cycle

The 24-hour diurnal rhythm which produces sleep at night and waking in the morning is driven by the suprachiasmatic nucleus of the hypothalamus. The sleep cycle itself is controlled by the pontine reticular formation. Recordings of sleep physiology with the polysomnogram (EEG, cardiac, respiratory, and eye-movement monitor) demonstrate a regular pattern of sleep cycles, at 90- to 100-minute intervals throughout the night. Figure 6-8 follows an individual through a typical night of sleep. Stages I through IV are progressively deeper levels of sleep, each characterized by a higher arousal threshold and greater synchronization (slowing) of brain electrical activity. After 40 to 50 minutes, the pattern is reversed, and the patient ascends to lighter sleep.

The next event is a 10- to 15-minute period of something dramatically different, rapid eye movement (REM) sleep. This stage is characterized by desynchronization of the EEG, fluttering movements of the eyes, postural relaxation, and autonomic changes (heart rate, respirations). When awakened at this point, patients often report that they are dreaming. Deprivation studies show that the REM phase of sleep

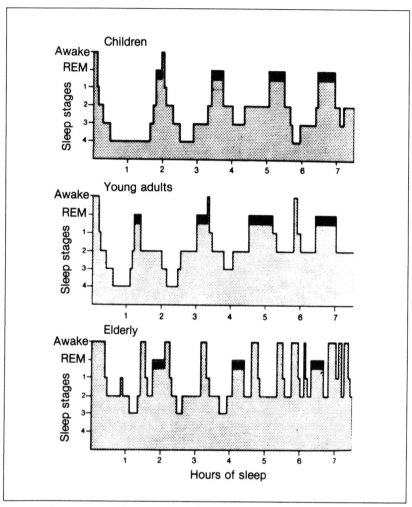

FIGURE 6-8. Sleep architecture. Rapid eye movement (REM) sleep alternates with non-rapid eye movement (NREM) in cycles approximating 90 minutes in all age groups. Delta sleep is prominent in childhood and decreases in the elderly as awakenings and wake times increase. (From A. Kales and J.D. Kales, Sleep disorders: Recent findings in the diagnosis and treatment of disturbed sleep. *N. Engl. J. Med.* 290 : 487, 1974, with permission.)

is independently necessary; sleep without it is not satisfying. Four or five REM intervals typically occur during the night.

Centers in the pontine reticular formation produce the sleep cycle. Lesions of the locus coeruleus, adjacent reticular formation, or dorsal raphe interfere with the cyclic alternation of REM and non-REM sleep. Relaxation of muscle tone during REM sleep requires descending inhibition of spinal reflexes. Structures in the medial pontine tegmentum are necessary if this is to occur. Hobson and McCarley propose a model in which reciprocal interaction of inhibitory centers (locus coeruleus, dorsal raphe) and excitatory centers (cholinergic nuclei in the pontine reticular formation) generates a 90-minute oscillation, and drives the events of the sleep cycle.

Sleep Disorders

Disturbances in sleep are fairly common. Patients may present with insomnia (too little sleep) or with excessive daytime sleepiness. The latter presentation can occur with *sleep apnea,* which deprives the nervous system of needed rest overnight, or with *narcolepsy,* a disorder of intrinsic sleep mechanisms. During World War I, an epidemic of encephalitis was described (encephalitis lethargica). This illness produced a prolonged, pathologic hypersomnolence (sleeping sickness). Today insomnia is a more prevalent phenomenon, as demonstrated by the range of prescription and nonprescription sedatives sold each year. In addition to drug therapy, there has been a proliferation of late-night television for the truly desperate.

The common cause of insomnia is anxiety or depression. The typical pattern is one of early-morning awakening. The patient may wake up at 3 or 4 A.M. to ruminate, and then be unable to get back to sleep. Pain is another frequent cause of insomnia. The pain pathway is highly interconnected with the brainstem reticular system, and traffic on this pathway tends to produce arousal. Alcohol and many sedative drugs interfere with normal sleep, and patients awaken tired. This is particularly true for the barbiturate sedatives, which depress REM sleep.

Abnormal Breathing During Sleep

Causes of excessive daytime sleepiness include the sleep apnea syndrome and its variations. In normal subjects, the physiology of breathing changes in deep sleep and REM sleep. Alterations are seen in the respiratory pattern and in the threshold for reflex responses to hypoxia and hypercapnia. For many patients, breathing problems during sleep are related to morbid obesity. Because of the increased mechanical work of breathing, these patients tend to hypoventilate. This difficulty is especially prominent during stage IV (slow wave) sleep. In addition, mechanical forces may collapse the upper airway at the level of the hypopharynx. Loud snoring is often a sign of inspiratory stridor in these patients. Patients may be roused, and do not get the full benefit of an uninterrupted sleep cycle. In some patients with sleep apnea, loss of muscle tone during REM sleep involves the upper airway and intercostals. A mixture of mechanisms may exist in the same patient, and weight loss alone is sometimes not sufficient to reverse the deficit.

Narcolepsy

Narcolepsy is the other principal cause of excessive daytime sleepiness. As the syndrome is defined clinically, there are four component parts: sleep attacks, cataplexy, sleep paralysis, and transition to sleep hallucinations. Not every patient will have all four. It is frightening for patients to awaken with paralysis, though symptoms pass in a few moments. Cataplexy is more disabling. It is a sudden lapse in muscle tone, which occurs during emotional moments (laughter, surprise, anger, even sexual intercourse). Patients fall or collapse, without loss of consciousness. The narcolepsy syndrome is described in families, and is probably determined by genetic mechanisms.

Studies of sleep physiology in narcolepsy show a very short latency before REM sleep appears. During REM sleep, there is normally inhibition of spinal reflexes and loss of muscle tone. The phenomena of cataplexy and sleep paralysis suggest an inappropriate activation of these mechanisms during the waking state. The broader hypothesis characterizes narcolepsy as a disorder of brainstem mechanisms for REM sleep control. A canine animal model has been described, in which postmortem analysis shows decreased turnover of dopamine and norepinephrine. There is also enhanced sensitivity of muscarinic cholinergic receptors in the pontine reticular formation. Tricyclic antidepressants stop cataplexy in human patients. Stimulant drugs are used to reduce sleep attacks.

BIBLIOGRAPHY

Hobson, J.A., and McCarley, R. The brain as a dream state generator. *Am. J. Psychiatry* 134 : 1335–1348, 1977.
Kales, A., Vela-Bueno, A., and Kales, J. Sleep disorders: sleep apnea and narcolepsy. *Ann. Intern. Med.* 106 : 434–443, 1987.
Klietman, N. *Sleep and Wakefulness.* Chicago: University of Chicago Press, 1965.
Mesulam, M. Attention, Confusional States, and Neglect. In M. Mesulam (ed.), *Principles of Behavioral Neurology.* Philadelphia: Davis, 1985.
Plum, F., and Posner, J. *The Diagnosis of Stupor and Coma* (3rd ed.). Philadelphia: Davis, 1980.
Popper, K.R., and Eccles, J.C. *The Self and Its Brain.* Heidelberg, West Germany: Springer-Verlag, 1981.

CHAPTER 7

Seizures

Seizures are described in the records of ancient civilizations. References to epileptic persons are found in the Code of Hammurabi. As recently as the nineteenth century, seizures were thought to impart spiritual qualities. Some of the mythology surrounding the epileptic is found in the writings of Dostoevski, himself afflicted with seizures. Vincent van Gogh had epilepsy, as did Alexander the Great. These men led productive lives in an era when anticonvulsant drugs were unavailable.

Seizures are relatively common in contemporary medical practice. Of young men who register for military service, just under 1 percent have a recorded history of seizures. The chance of having a seizure at some point during life is 2 to 5 percent. This surprising figure includes the risk of a single febrile seizure during childhood. Most seizures do not recur, and are related to some metabolic or environmental circumstance. About 0.5 percent of the population have seizures repeatedly; only these persons are said to have epilepsy.

A seizure is a temporary disturbance of brain electrical activity, an event associated with a brief alteration in nervous system function. Underlying the paroxysm is a *synchronized depolarization* of neurons. The clinical expression of a seizure is often quite dramatic. During a generalized seizure, the patient has spasm and jerking of the limbs, loss of consciousness, and incontinence (involuntary loss of urine). For a partial seizure, the manifestations are more subtle.

DEFINITION, RECOGNITION, SEIZURE TYPE DESCRIPTION

The recognition of a typical grand mal (generalized) seizure poses little challenge, but sometimes the diagnosis of a seizure event requires a careful history or a few moments of observation, or both. A seizure must be distinguished from other disorders that result in transient disturbance of brain function, such as syncope, concussion, or a transient ischemic attack. Episodes of hyperventilation, breath holding, or panic attacks sometimes simulate partial seizures. The same patient may have both real seizures and hysterical seizures (pseudoseizures). The hallmarks of a typical seizure are (1) brief duration, most typically 1 or 2 minutes, (2) deviation of the head and eyes during an event, (3) jerking of the limbs or automatic behavior, (4) disturbance of consciousness, (5) tongue biting or incontinence, (6) a period of confusion in the subsequent minutes, and (7) a period of amnesia for the events of the seizure. Some of these typical features are absent in a partial, or restricted seizure. For any given patient, seizure manifestations tend to be stereotypic: consecutive episodes are almost identical. Some patients have more than one seizure type.

Seizures are classified into two principal categories according to their electrophysiologic pattern and clinical expression. The classification of the epilepsies is summarized in Table 7-1. A seizure disorder is said to be partial if it is restricted, a regional disturbance of cerebral activity. It is a generalized seizure if the whole brain participates. Partial seizures are subdivided further into partial simple and partial complex, *according to whether consciousness is disturbed*. A *partial simple seizure* is a focal motor or focal sensory disturbance, with the patient awake and alert. *Partial complex seizures* cause a brief lapse of consciousness or staring spell. An aura or warning is often present before a partial complex seizure, sometimes involving olfaction. Some patients describe an odd emotional state, a feeling of apprehension, familiarity (déjà vu), or depersonalization. Amnesia and confusion are common. Automatisms, such as smacking of the lips, may be observed. Partial complex seizures are sometimes called *temporal lobe epilepsy*, as the limbic system structures in the anterior temporal lobe are most often involved. (Twenty to forty percent originate from the adjacent orbital frontal or occipital lobe.)

A *primary generalized seizure* is a whole-brain dysrhythmia. The commonest such disorder is the *tonic-clonic* (grand mal) seizure. The patient will fall to the ground unconscious, rigid, and cyanotic for 15 to 20 seconds (tonic phase), and may salivate or lose control of the sphincters. This is followed by rhythmic contractions of the limbs for another 30 to 40 seconds (clonic phase). Consciousness recovers slowly over the next several minutes, though the patient is often sleepy and confused (postictal) for an hour or more. There are also various kinds of nonconvulsive generalized seizures, the most common of which is the *primary absence*, or petit mal. This is a disorder of childhood and adolescence. During the 2- to 10-second absence, or staring spell, the patient may have eye blinks. The spell is associated with a 3-cps, generalized spike and slow wave discharge on the elec-

TABLE 7-1. Classification of Seizure Disorders

I. Primary generalized seizures
   A. Tonic-clonic (grand mal)
   B. Primary absence (petit mal)
   C. Myoclonic
   D. Juvenile atonic and myoclonic
   E. Infantile spasms
II. Partial seizures
   A. Partial simple (consciousness is maintained), focal motor, sensory, jacksonian seizures
   B. Partial complex (disturbance of consciousness), temporolimbic epilepsy
   C. Secondary generalized seizures

troencephalogram (EEG). A variety of *atonic* and *myoclonic* seizure types occur, most typically in childhood. Some patients have *reflex epilepsy*, seizures that are triggered by a specific activity or stimulus, such as laughing, reading, or flashing light.

A partial seizure can spread to trigger a generalized seizure. This event is called a *secondary generalized seizure*. The jacksonian seizure, a partial seizure which begins discretely, distally in a limb, commonly does this. As the discharge migrates along the cortical map (homunculus), other limb muscles are recruited. People observe aghast, as the seizure "marches" across the body. A generalized seizure with loss of consciousness may ensue. The distinction between a primary generalized seizure and a partial seizure with secondary spread is often difficult. Careful EEG and behavioral observations during a seizure are sometimes required to make the distinction.

In addition to a seizure type description, it is important to have information about the etiology or cause of the patient's seizures. The patient's prognosis is most closely related to the underlying cause of the seizures. Many different diseases affecting the nervous system, toxins, and metabolic disorders can cause a seizure. A partial list is found in Table 7-2. Sometimes the cause of a generalized seizure is not found, and the seizure disorder is said to be idiopathic.

In this context, it is important to remember that the ability to support a seizure is a property of the normal brain. With its intricate network of excitatory interactions, the vertebrate cortex has a built-in predisposition for synchronized discharges. The brain of any higher animal can generate a seizure when stimulated by electric shock. Likewise, seizures occur when a toxin or abnormal metabolic environment favors neuronal irritability and depolarization. (Alcohol and cocaine are particularly common offenders.)

TABLE 7-2. Causes of Seizures

Congenital or perinatal disorder
Infectious
  Meningitis
  Encephalitis
  Cortical vein thrombosis, cerebral abscess
Trauma
  Closed head injury with cerebral contusion
  Penetrating wound
Neoplasm
  Primary brain tumor
  Metastatic cancer
Vascular
  Arteriovenous malformation
  Cerebral infarction
  Parenchymal or subarachnoid hemorrhage
Metabolic
  Electrolyte abnormality (esp. hypocalcemia), uremia, hypoglycemia,
    hepatic failure
Toxins
  Alcohol withdrawal
  Cocaine
  Other substance abuse
Mesial-temporal sclerosis
Simple febrile convulsion
Idiopathic

CELLULAR MECHANISM OF EPILEPSY

In the last 25 to 30 years, it has been possible to investigate the physiologic events which underlie a seizure. The production of even a partial seizure involves synchronized activity in a large area of the brain. In between seizure events, in the interictal period, a regional disturbance can be recorded in patients with partial epilepsy. This *interictal discharge*, a burst of synchronized firing in a few thousand neurons, is active even though seizures are not occurring. Several model systems exist to study epileptiform discharges. Synchronized firing can be recorded from clusters of nerve cells in tissue culture, or from an isolated slice of hippocampus. To a large degree, our understanding of seizure mechanisms derives from recordings of the interictal discharge from the neocortex or hippocampus of animals with partial seizures. (Primary generalized epilepsy is considered separately.)

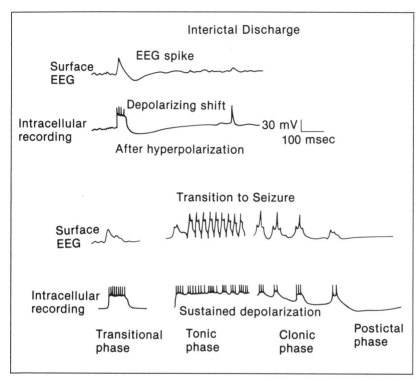

FIGURE 7-1. Top figure shows the interictal discharge. When the surface EEG records a spike discharge, a local population of neurons has undergone a depolarizing shift (DS). This is reflected in the intracellular recording. At the crest of the DS, a rapid burst of action potentials is observed. A period of hyperpolarization and decreased activity follows. Bottom figure illustrates the transition to seizure. The afterhyperpolarization is replaced by a depolarization. Protracted trains of action potentials develop. The surface EEG changes from simple spikes to complex, polyphasic spikes. Widely synchronized cortical activity results in a tonic-clonic seizure. (Modified from A.L. Pearlman and R.C. Collins, *Neurological Pathophysiology* [3rd ed.]. New York: Oxford, 1984, p. 234.)

Interictal Discharge: The Depolarizing Shift

The interictal discharge is the product of synchronized depolarization and firing in a group of neurons. It is a population event, an abnormal collective behavior of neurons. Intracellular recording from a single neuron within the epileptic focus shows a characteristic disturbance, the paroxysmal depolarizing shift (DS, Fig. 7-1). The DS is a large-amplitude (20–50 mV), sustained wave of depolarization, a regional phenomenon lasting 70 to 150 msec. Superimposed on the crest of the wave are bursts of high-frequency action potentials. If enough neurons participate, this event can be recorded in surface electrodes as an EEG spike. In the subsequent 0.5 to 1.5 seconds, a period of hyperpolarization and relative inexcitability follows, sometimes called the *afterhyperpolarization*.

Under normal conditions, the neuron's membrane potential is determined by ion concentration gradients. There are voltage-dependent channels along the membrane for cations; fluxes in these ions propagate the action potential. At the synapse, ligand-gated channels specific for Na^+, K^+, or Cl^- induce a barrage of postsynaptic potentials. The channel at the N-methyl-d-aspartate (NMDA)–type glutamate receptor, when opened, is permeable to calcium as well as sodium. The typical excitatory postsynaptic potential (EPSP) is 2 to 10 mV in amplitude, less than 20 msec in duration. What combination of events could trigger the DS, a larger and more sustained depolarization?

Factors Favoring Instability

Cortical structures contain a number of built-in, positive feedback mechanisms which could potentially contribute to instability and synchronized bursting. Foremost among these is the preponderance of excitatory synaptic interactions. Neural network models suggest that nerve cell populations in which excitatory links predominate develop a tendency to synchronized firing. Computer models of cortical networks may provide an ideal environment in which to study the phenomenon of epileptogenesis.

Ionic changes in the environment of the epileptic focus also contribute to its instability. Potassium is increased in the extracellular fluid, as high as 8 to 12 mM during a discharge, while calcium concentrations are decreased by 50 percent. An increase in extracellular potassium concentration tends to depolarize the membrane. During the DS and ensuing action potential, further release of potassium occurs.

Cortical neurons have small afterpotentials, and are thus capable of rapid firing. Recordings from the exposed cortex of patients during neurosurgical procedures have shown discharge rates of up to 900 per second in a seizure focus. In addition, there is a form of high-frequency or *use-dependent potentiation* which occurs in cortical circuits. These factors favor burst firing.

The NMDA receptor channel is another source of potential mischief in cortical circuits. When activated under physiologic conditions, it is blocked by magnesium, but it can pop open as the cell depolarizes.

When open, the NMDA receptor channel carries a large calcium and sodium ion current, enhancing the tendency toward depolarization. NMDA receptors are found in greatest abundance in the hippocampus, the cortex with the lowest seizure threshold.

Stabilizing Influences

Countervailing forces oppose the tendency toward explosive activation of cortical neurons. These cells contain a calcium-dependent potassium channel, a fail-safe mechanism which can oppose the depolarizing force of an inward calcium current. The greatest constraint on uncontrolled activation of cortical circuits is the deployment of synaptic inhibition.

Recurrent (feedback) inhibition helps to maintain the afterhyperpolarization that follows the DS. Hyperpolarization can also be recorded from a regional neighborhood of the focus, and helps to contain the discharge. The neocortex is heavily populated with inhibitory local circuit neurons. This neuronal population uses γ-aminobutyric acid (GABA) as its predominant neurotransmitter type. GABA-mediated inhibition opens chloride channels to generate the inhibitory postsynaptic potential (IPSP), usually associated with a slight hyperpolarization. Large cortical neurons have axon collaterals, many of which influence inhibitory interneurons nearby. The local circuit thus sets up an inhibitory surround adjacent to an active discharge (Fig. 7-2). The phenomenon of regional inhibition, well studied in the physiology of other cortical systems, acts as a natural containment mechanism to terminate the discharge and limit its spread.

What Initiates the DS?

The DS is a complex phenomenon, whose triggering mechanism is not fully understood. Unstable or inherently irritable neurons may initiate the discharge. Other hypotheses consider changes in the regional metabolic milieu or local synaptic interactions. Many experts believe that the depolarizing shift is a synaptic event.

One hypothesis holds that the DS is a postsynaptic potential, amplified by slow calcium currents. The initial event might involve a convergence of excitatory inputs (or some membrane defect), opening ion channels, and allowing sodium (and calcium) to enter from the extracellular space. Calcium influx occurs through voltage-gated calcium channels, ultimately through the channel at the NMDA receptor. As the depolarization develops, more and more ion channels are opened.

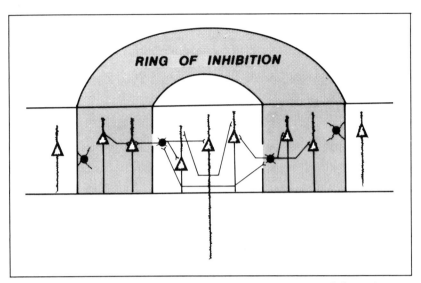

FIGURE 7-2. Depolarization of cortical neuron in the center of the active seizure focus tends to recruit neighboring cells, via excitatory recurrent connections. When inhibitory local circuit neurons (black stellate cells) are activated, they promote a ring of inhibition. Surrounding inhibition helps to contain the seizure discharge. In addition, these cells inhibit activity within the seizure focus, contributing to the afterhyperpolarization. (Adapted from A. Pearlman and R.C. Collins, Neurological Pathophysiology (3rd ed.). New York: Oxford University Press, 1984.)

The slow calcium current acts as a positive feedback mechanism to sustain the depolarization. Given the concentration gradient for calcium across the membrane, a moderate (20–30 mV) and somewhat prolonged depolarization can develop. In response, *calcium-gated potassium channels* eventually open and allow a repolarizing potassium current out into the extracellular space. This second-stage response presumably terminates the depolarizing shift and initiates the afterhyperpolarization.

An important aspect of the DS is occurrence of multiple, high-frequency action potentials on the crest of the slow depolarizing wave. Cortical neurons that reach threshold during the DS commence high-frequency firing. The synchronization of the DS is thought to be the product of local synaptic interactions. A kind of positive feedback is generated by the network of excitatory connections, which promotes the regional spread of the DS. In addition, a large field potential is generated in the cortex by depolarization of the vertically oriented pyramidal cells, conducting through the medium of extracellular fluids. This electrical field also encourages the spread of the depolarization.

Transition to Seizure

The events which mark the transition from interictal discharge to seizure are also illustrated in Figure 7-1. With time, the afterhyperpolarization begins to diminish in size, and then disappears altogether, ultimately to be replaced by a modest *depolarization*. It is unclear what factors promote this drift. High-frequency firing appears to cause potentiation at excitatory cortical synapses, while inhibitory synaptic mechanisms appear to show frequency-related fatigue (depression). An increase in the extracellular potassium concentration alters resting membrane potential. The induced drift in membrane potential serves to prolong the DS, and increases the tendency toward cell firing. The end result is a more sustained depolarization, persisting over several seconds. This discharge overwhelms the local inhibitory containment mechanisms, and recruits other neurons in synchronized firing. The discharge may spread in this manner to contiguous areas, or to other homologous regions via long corticocortical connections. Seizure activity beginning focally can spread to the contralateral cerebral hemisphere via the corpus callosum. Some investigators believe that synchronization of the hemispheres occurs through the participation of a subcortical projection system, a network of brainstem and thalamocortical connections.

After 20 to 30 seconds of repeated firing, the tonic phase of a generalized seizure, cell bursting becomes intermittent. After 1 to 2 minutes of active discharge, inhibitory mechanisms are sufficiently engaged to promote a sustained hyperpolarization and postictal depression. The participating parts of the nervous system become relatively inexcitable for a period of time that ranges from several minutes to hours. Release and accumulation of inhibitory amino acid and peptide neurotransmitters is thought to be important in the physiology of the postictal depression.

Toward a More General Theory of Epileptogenesis

How is the epileptic focus different from normal brain? The events of the interictal discharge are local phenomena. As reviewed, the depolarizing shift may be due to overactivity of local excitatory synaptic interactions or to a regional deficiency of inhibition. Giant synaptic potentials resembling the depolarizing shift have been observed when the chloride channel is blocked and the NMDA receptor mechanism is activated. Drugs which block the $GABA_A$ receptor are universally active as convulsants. A decrease in GABA synaptic markers has been noted in immunohistochemical studies of chronic epileptic foci, suggesting that the delicate balance between excitation and synaptic inhibition may be altered after injury.

Another hypothesis suggests that regional metabolic disturbances foster the depolarizing shift. Glial cells have an active role in maintaining the potassium ion concentration in the extracellular space, and mopping up excess neurotransmitter fragments. Local abnormalities in the neuron's metabolic milieu may account for the instability and shift in membrane potential. A rather different theory of epileptogenesis blames the "damaged neuron." Perhaps an ultrastructural or membrane disturbance in some of the large pyramidal neurons in a cortical structure favors instability and engenders the depolarizing shift. As there are numerous different causes of seizure events, it is unrealistic to expect to find a unitary mechanism. All of these factors may be at work within a single focus.

Primary Generalized Seizures: The Role of the Thalamocortical Projection System

Some seizure events appear to involve the whole brain from the instant of onset. Penfield and Jasper proposed in the 1940s that structures in the brainstem and diencephalon play an active role in synchronizing the whole-brain dysrhythmia in these patients. This has been known since as the *centrencephalic theory*. Penfield observed that low-frequency stimulation of the intralaminar and reticular thalamic nuclei, part of the "diffuse thalamocortical projection system," would evoke a 3-cps spike and wave discharge similar to those recorded during petit mal epilepsy. A hypothesis suggests that this recticulo-thalamocortical network resonates at 3 cps. It is not clear at present to what degree the thalamus and other subcortical structures act to synchronize bursting and coordinate the clinical expression of a grand mal seizure. Studies of regional metabolic activity with 2-deoxyglucose in animals with generalized epilepsy indicate that parts of the thalamus, the mammillary nucleus of the hypothalamus, and the substantia nigra are active during a seizure.

THE ELECTROENCEPHALOGRAM

Much maligned and certainly misunderstood, the EEG is a technique for recording cerebral activity. For clinical purposes, it is impractical to

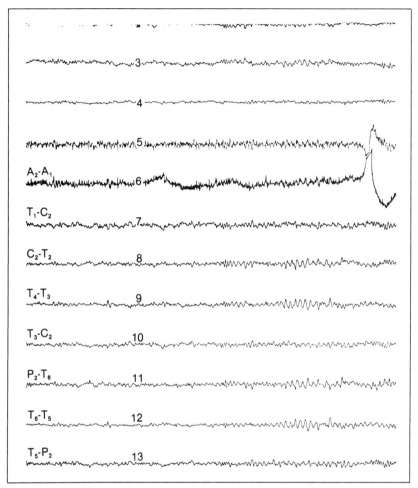

FIGURE 7-3. Normal EEG. The record shows a normal mixture of cerebral background activity. In the posterior channels, 8-cps (alpha) rhythm can be observed. Mark denotes 1 second.

sample brain electrical activity with penetrating electrodes. The EEG was invented by Hans Berger in 1929 as a method of recording cerebral activity through the cranial vault and scalp. The modern EEG uses 20 silver-plated electrodes, applied to the scalp with collodion or paste. Eight (or 16) electrode pairs are connected through independent amplifier channels, and each channel has its output connected to a recording pen. The patient is monitored in various states over a 40- to 80-minute interval, as different combinations of electrodes are sampled. The technique is sensitive to many different kinds of recording artifact, and the record is notoriously difficult to interpret (Fig. 7-3).

The "brain waves" are generated by membrane potentials of cortical neurons, principally the apical dendrites of the large pyramidal cells. In these large cell surface membranes, the ionic currents are big enough to create a dipole which can be detected through the scalp. This is similar to the process of recording electrocardiographic activity through the chest wall. The depolarization of heart muscle fibers is synchronized, so that large waves of current are generated. The cerebral cortex, on the other hand, processes billions of independent synaptic events and the surface electrode sees only a moving average. Intuitively, you would expect the deflections of the pen to reflect the action potential and cell-firing events. In fact, however, most of the recorded activity is generated by EPSPs and IPSPs in pyramidal neurons, beneath the threshold for cell firing. Background cerebral activity so recorded is analyzed by decomposing the complex waveform into frequency components, or intrinsic rhythms. The 8- to 12-cps activity is salient in posterior leads during waking; this activity is known as the alpha rhythm. Large amounts of 1- to 3-cps, or delta, activity in a waking patient indicate an underlying abnormality.

How Does the EEG Look at Seizures?

The synchronized firing of a large population of cortical neurons is an electrical event big enough to cause a sharp transient deflection, or spike, in the surface recording. Most of the work done with the EEG in seizure patients focuses on the detection of the interictal discharge (Fig. 7-4). The sensitivity of the test, looking for paroxysmal discharges in the interictal record, is only moderate. Perhaps 60 percent of patients with new-onset epilepsy will have a spike or a suspicious sharp deflection of some kind on the interictal EEG. Often the abnormalities recorded (excess regional slowing, bursts of generalized 4–7-cps activity) are of a nonspecific nature. Enhancements in the recording technique increase the yield in diagnosis. If partial complex seizures of temporal lobe origin are suspected, recording is often done in transition to sleep. The yield is increased further if sphenoidal or nasopharyngeal electrodes are used, as the medial temporal lobe is quite far from the scalp, and considerable signal attenuation occurs during volume conduction.

The most useful information derives from recording the patient during a seizure. A seizure is an infrequent event for most patients, and a 40-minute sampling is unlikely to capture one. Nonetheless, for some kinds of management decisions a look at the ictal record is most helpful. Telemetry, remote monitoring of the EEG signal over a prolonged interval, is used for this purpose. EEG recorded by telemetry

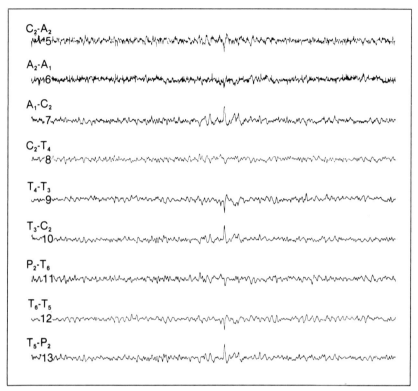

FIGURE 7-4. EEG record from a patient with partial epilepsy, showing an interictal discharge (spike). The spike can be seen to reverse polarity about the site of origin of the discharge, near the T3 electrode.

during a generalized seizure is shown in Figure 7-5. The seizure can be seen to begin focally, with secondary generalization. Combined EEG and behavioral observations of the patient during a seizure are the best data for studying the physiology of the patient's seizure disorder, especially when multiple foci are present. Unfortunately, telemetry is costly and is generally reserved for problem cases.

ANIMAL MODELS OF EPILEPSY

Animal models are essential to the study of seizure mechanisms in the laboratory. Most mammals have seizure phenomena sufficiently like human epilepsy to be of some interest. Several animal species have spontaneous seizures, like the primary generalized seizures that occur in human patients. Having an animal model allows experimentation,

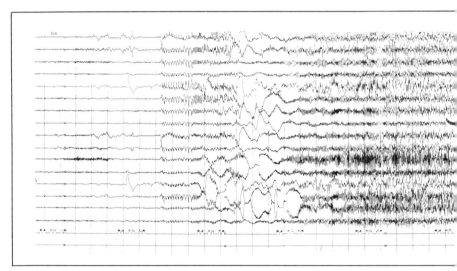

FIGURE 7-5. The ictal record: EEG recording of a patient during a tonic-clonic seizure. Seizure begins with a rhythmic high-frequency discharge, followed by multiple, closely grouped spikes of variable amplitude (tonic phase). This period, lasting generally 10 to 30 seconds, is followed by distinct polyspikes, separated by isoelectric periods (correlated with the clonic phase). A postictal period of relative inexcitability and flat background follows. (Courtesy of John Ives, Neurology Department, Beth Israel Hospital, Boston.)

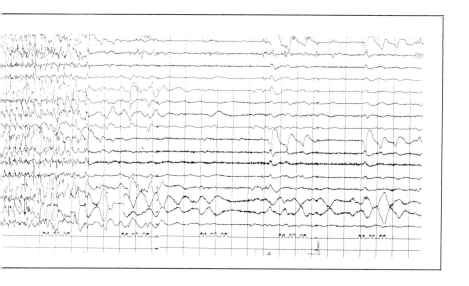

and fosters the examination of new ideas about epileptogenesis and seizure control. A more important practical consequence is a laboratory environment for studying the action of antiepileptic drugs.

The most robust animal model for seizure phenomena is created by applying an irritant substance to the cortex. This process establishes a cortical focus, suitable for studying partial simple and secondary generalized seizures. The traditional method involves direct application of alumina gel onto the pial membrane. Penicillin is also a convulsant, when applied directly to the cortex in very high local concentration. These techniques have been useful in the study of focal seizure mechanisms, though the epileptic activity so induced in the rat or cat does not persist over weeks. There have been several efforts to mimic the chronic persistent focus observed with cerebral contusion by freeze-injuring the cortex or by deposition of metals into the tissue. Most seizure activity produced by these techniques diminishes over time but persists long enough to study the influence of antiepileptic drugs on the interictal discharge.

To study primary generalized seizures in an animal model, a different approach is required. Maximal electric shock (electroconvulsive therapy, ECT) can be used to induce a generalized seizure, to test the anticonvulsant properties of a new drug. Systematic administration of phenylenetetrazole or high-dose penicillin in the cat will induce generalized epilepsy, with a spike and slow wave discharge recorded from scalp electrodes. This is the laboratory model most appropriate to the study of petit mal. Antagonists of GABA synaptic function such as bicuculine cause a variety of generalized convulsive and nonconvulsive seizures. These drugs interfere with inhibitory mechanisms which restrain the spread of seizure discharges in the cortex, as reviewed above.

A number of single gene mutations and metabolic disorders have been encountered which result in spontaneous seizure activity. At this date, at least 14 single gene mutations have been associated with epilepsy in the mouse. One such mutant, the totterer, has been found to have a disorder of noradrenergic neurons. There is generalized overgrowth of noradrenergic nerve terminals with excess synaptic availability of norepinephrine. Another mouse mutant has been identified with myoclonic activity, in relation to an isolated disorder of the glycine synapse. These animal mutants provide a medium for studying the cellular expression of inherited epilepsies, and for learning how cortical excitability is modified by alterations at the molecular level.

Amygdaloid Kindling: A Model for Temporolimbic Epilepsy

Certain structures in the vertebrate nervous system exhibit a tendency toward spontaneous seizures after occasional, subconvulsive electrical stimulation, a phenomenon known as *kindling*. The amygdala has a low seizure threshold and is remarkably sensitive to seizure induction by this technique. Amygdaloid kindling is often considered a model for human partial complex seizures, many of which arise from limbic system structures within the medial temporal lobe.

Kindling occurs from the repeated administration of a subconvulsive electrical stimulus, delivered at regular intervals. A 60-Hz stimulus, applied for 1 second, is sufficient to induce a brief depolarization, or afterdischarge. The same stimulus is readministered after a rest interval according to some fixed schedule; daily electrical stimulation for 1 second at a time is commonly employed. Within days stimulation will begin to evoke a more prolonged afterdischarge, soon accompanied by a clinical event. A regular sequence of seizure phenomena is observed as the response grows: initially facial clonus, later head-nodding, limb-twitching, and rearing-up. Ultimately the animal will fall over unresponsive as a full secondary generalized seizure is kindled. At the final stage, after several weeks of daily stimulation, the focus will exhibit spontaneous seizure activity that is independent of stimulation, and the kindling effect is generally persistent. The olfactory bulb, entorhinal cortex, globus pallidus, septal area, and hippocampus can also be kindled, though amygdaloid kindling is perhaps the easiest to effect and the most durable.

The phenomenon is a model for partial complex seizure disorders in man, with some startling clinical implications. The kindled focus in the amygdala (or in some cortical structure) represents a persistent modification of neuronal function. Though the morphologic basis for this change is not understood, it is evident that the brain can "learn" to have a seizure. Within these regions, an epileptic disorder can establish itself, or even spread to involve other contiguous or highly connected regions. This phenomenon is observed in some human patients with temporolimbic epilepsy. Over a period of years, a temporal lobe focus will sometimes elicit activity in the contralateral temporal lobe: a "mirror focus." With time, the mirror focus may become capable of supporting independent seizure activity. At this point, resection of the focus in the temporal lobe on the symptomatic side may no longer cure the patient of his or her seizures.

MECHANISM OF ACTION OF ANTIEPILEPTIC DRUGS

Studies in animal models help to understand and predict the clinical effect of seizure medications. The commonly used drugs have differing effects on aspects of the interictal discharge, transition, and spread of paroxysmal activity. Patients with various types of seizure disorders also show different patterns of response to medications.

TABLE 7-3. Efficacy of Commonly Used
Antiepileptic Drugs in Animal Models of Epilepsy*

	Animal Model		
Drug	Alumina Gel Focus	Phenylenetetrazole	Amygdaloid Kindling
Phenytoin	+++		
Valproate	++	+++	?
Ethosuximide		+++	
Carbamazepine	+++		+++
Phenobarbital	+++	++	++

*The ability of various drugs to control experimental epilepsy is graded, ranging from
no entry (no control) to ++++ (very effective control). These studies are somewhat
predictive of the success of drugs in controlling human seizure disorders.

Some of the variation is individual, and all too often the efficacy of
antiepileptic drugs is limited by side effects. Even so, the therapeutic
effect of a drug on the principal seizure types is to some degree
predictable, based on animal studies. Table 7-3 reviews the efficacy of
five commonly used drugs in three different animal models of the
epilepsies.

    Petit mal seizures do not respond well to phenytoin, as the animal
work would predict. Rather, this form of primary generalized seizure
disorder is best treated with ethosuximide or valproic acid. Valproate
is useful in many of the generalized epilepsies of childhood and early
adult life. Partial simple and secondary generalized seizures respond
equally well to phenytoin, phenobarbital, or carbamazepine. While
any of these drugs may be effective in partial complex seizures of
temporal lobe origin, phenytoin does not inhibit the experimental
kindling phenomenon. For purely theoretical reasons, carbamazepine
may be preferable for limiting the evolution of the mirror focus.
Because there are fewer effects on cognition with its long-term use,
carbamazepine is preferred by many epilepsy specialists as the drug
of choice for focal seizures.

Mechanism of Action at a Cellular Level

Several of the commonly used antiepileptic drugs effect GABA-mediated
synaptic inhibition in cortical structures. The barbiturate and benzodi-
azepine drugs appear to exert their effect on the GABA receptor complex. These agents act indirectly to enhance the binding affinity for
GABA at its receptor. By enhancing the physiologic effect of GABA,
these drugs potentiate regional synaptic inhibition. Inhibitory mech-

anisms limit the spread of paroxysmal depolarization, as discussed above. The pharmacologic effect of these drugs appears to favor the containment of the seizure discharge. Too much GABA-mediated inhibition in the neocortex, however, can limit normal nervous system functions. These categories of antiepileptic drugs share the potential for causing sedation when present in excessive amounts.

The mechanism of action of phenytoin appears to be different and somewhat more complex. In stressed, excitable tissues, phenytoin appears to suppress repetitive firing. High-frequency bursting is a property of cortical neurons which contributes to seizure formation. The critical effect of phenytoin on high-frequency activity appears to be a function of its influence on the membrane Na^+ channel. During high-frequency firing, phenytoin causes a block in the membrane's voltage-dependent Na^+ conductance. This effect on the Na^+ channel reduces the amplitude and rate of rise of the action potential. The net effect is an attenuation of high-frequency firing. Carbamazepine and valproic acid may have similar effects on high-frequency firing, though less is known about the mechanism of action of these drugs on epileptic irritability.

Treatment of Refractory Cases

The object of treatment is to eliminate seizures, especially grand mal seizures without warning. Other goals include single agent therapy, elimination of drug-related side effects, and full occupational and social rehabilitation. Of adult patients with partial complex and/or secondary generalized seizures, 20 to 40 percent fail to meet these treatment goals. For some of these patients, surgical removal of an established and treatment-resistant epileptic focus is an option.

BIBLIOGRAPHY

Brown, T., and Feldman, R. (eds). *Epilepsy: Diagnosis and Management*. Boston: Little, Brown, 1983.
Delgado-Escueta, A., et al. (eds.). Basic mechanism of the epilepsies: A symposium. *Ann. Neurol.* 16 (Suppl); 1984.
Dichter, M.A. The Epilepsies and Convulsive Disorders. In E. Braunwald, et al. (eds), *Principles of Internal Medicine* (11th ed.). New York: McGraw-Hill, 1987. Pp. 1921–1930.
Dichter, M.A., and Ayala, G.F. Cellular mechanisms of epilepsy: A status report. *Science* 237 : 157–164, 1987.
Pedley, T. The pathophysiology of focal epilepsy: Neurophysiological considerations. *Ann. Neurol.* 3 : 2–9, 1978.
Prince, D. Neurophysiology of epilepsy. *Annu. Rev. Neurosci.* 1 : 395–415, 1978.
Schwartzkroin, P., and Wyler, A. Mechanisms underlying epileptiform burst discharge. *Ann. Neurol.* 7 : 95–107, 1980.

CHAPTER 8

Cortical Function and Behavioral Neurology

The cerebral cortex is a relative newcomer in the evolutionary sense. The term refers to the mantle of gray matter that covers the cerebral hemispheres in higher animals (Fig. 8-1). *Neocortex* is distinguished from phylogenetically older cortical structures (the dorsal ridge of the reptile, the mammalian hippocampus) by its six-layered architecture. Neocortical area and mass have enlarged enormously with mammalian evolution. Many vertebrate biologists and paleontologists consider brain volume to be a crude marker of evolutionary achievement. Careful studies of comparative anatomy indicate that the development of neocortex relative to brainstem structures is better correlated with an animal's mental and behavioral complexity.

Enormous growth in cortical area is effected in advanced species by folding. Folding allows an expansion of the cortical mass without the necessity for any basic change in the pattern of vertical organization. In man the neocortex is spread over a surface area of 4,000 sq cm. Current estimates suggest a neuronal population of about 50 billion nerve cells in the adult (after greater than 50% attrition which occurs by the end of the first year of life). The cellular thickness of neocortex is relatively constant at 110 neurons per 30-μm-diameter column. In comparative studies by Powell and co-workers, the cellular content of a cortical column does not vary much across the evolutionary spectrum. The actual depth of cortex is greater in primates, due to an expanded volume of neuropil and richer dendritic arbor. But overall, encephalization in higher animals has been accomplished by enlargement of cortical surface area, without a dramatic change in the columnar architecture.

A further observation about cortical evolution derives from an analysis of the functional types of cortex and their distribution (Fig. 8-2). Primary sensory and motor cortex have enlarged only moderately as we ascend the phylogenetic scale. Much of the newest cortex is classified as association type. It is not dedicated to sensory processing or to

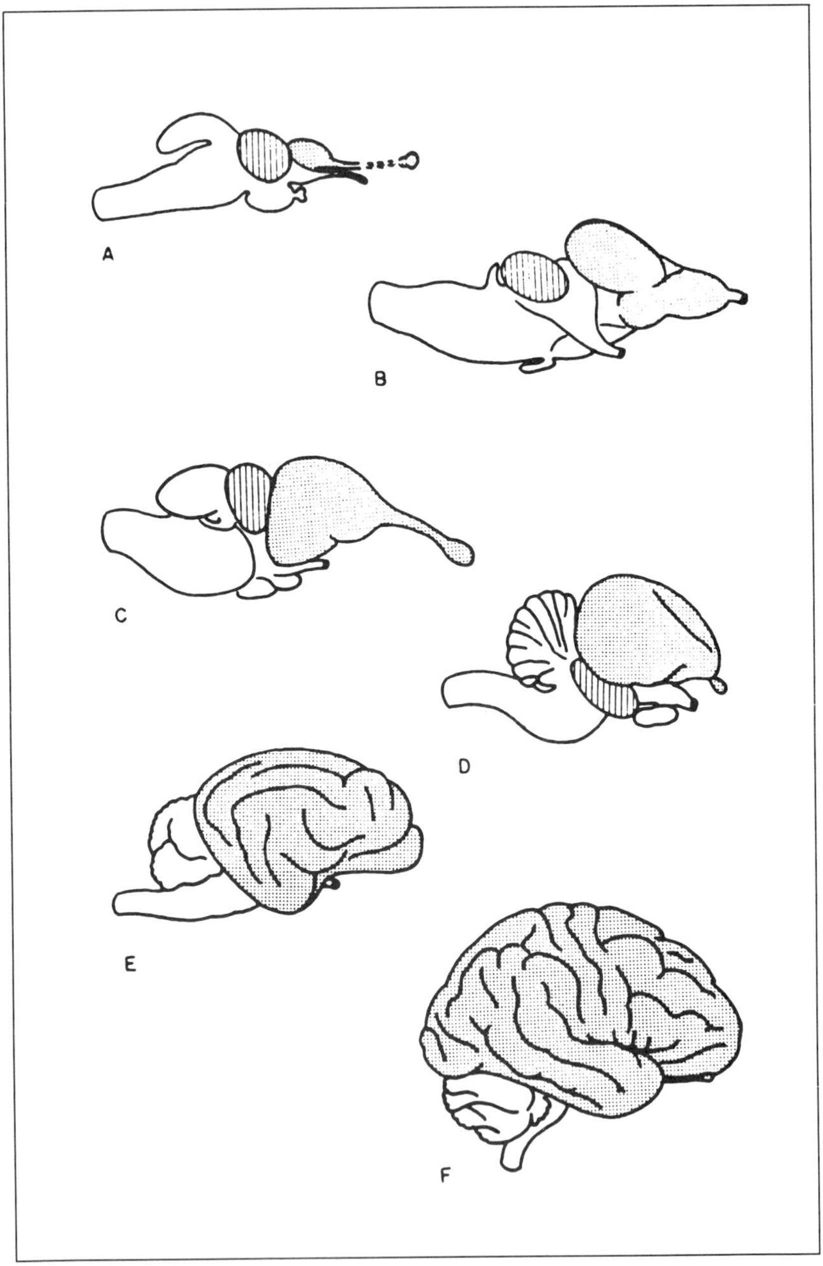

FIGURE 8-1. Stippled area denotes cerebral cortex, or its equivalent, which increases in relative size as we "ascend" the phylogenetic scale. Drawings are of different scale for the codfish (A), frog (B), alligator (C), pigeon (D), cat (E), and man (F). Vertical line shading indicates the optic tectum. (Reproduced from the *Neurosciences, 2nd Study Program* 1970, p. 12, by copyright permission of the Rockefeller University Press.)

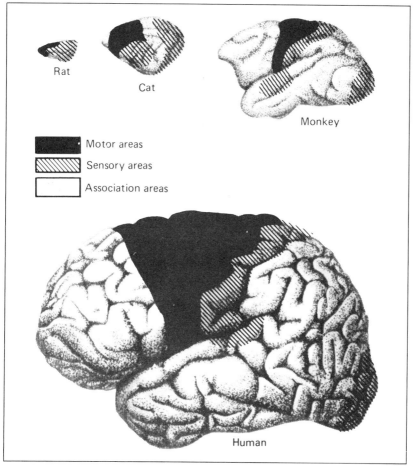

FIGURE 8-2. This drawing indicates the relative size of cortical areas in four mammals. Note the enormous enlargement in the primate of association cortex. (From E.R. Kandel and J.H. Schwartz, *Principles of Neural Science* [2nd ed.]. New York: Elsevier, 1985, p. 675, with permission.)

motor programming; most of its extrinsic connections derive from other cortex. Association cortex is thus able to pursue more complex and creative information processing. Expansion of the multimodal association cortex in the posterior parietal lobe and the frontal lobe is the most evident structural accomplishment of the human brain.

FUNCTIONAL ORGANIZATION

There are three types of cerebral cortex, sometimes designated as archicortex, paleocortex, and neocortex. Archicortex is the most primitive

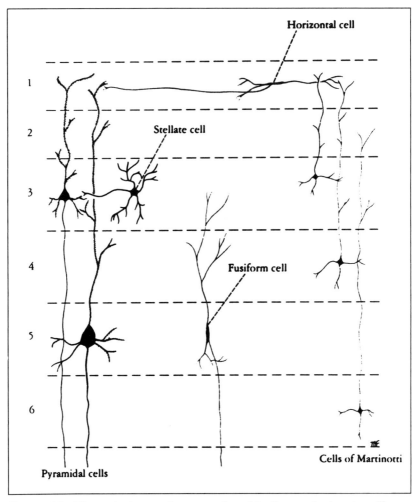

FIGURE 8-3. The main types of neurons found in the cerebral cortex. (From R. Snell, *Clinical Neuroanatomy for Medical Students* [2nd ed.]. Boston: Little, Brown, 1987, p. 284, with permission.)

cortex found in the human forebrain. Examples include the hippocampus, a rolled, three-layered structure, and the hippocampal remnant (indusium griseum), found adjacent to the corpus callosum. Paleocortex is a transitional cortical type, best exemplified by the entorhinal cortex of the temporal lobe. The cingulate gyrus is another transitional cortex; it is also a part of the limbic system.

Neocortex has a six-layered structure. Its principal cell types are shown in Figure 8-3. The pyramidal cells have upward-oriented apical

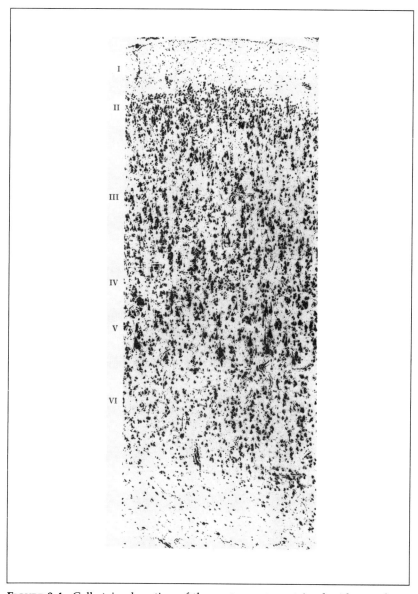

FIGURE 8-4. Cell-stained section of the motor cortex, stained with cresyl violet, of a human at 2 years of age. The six cortical layers can be distinguished by cell size and packing density. Note the giant pyramidal cells in layer V. (Reprinted by permission from J.L. Conel, *The Post Natal Development of the Cerebral Cortex.* Cambridge, Mass.: Harvard University Press, 1959. Vol. 6.)

dendrites, and large cell bodies, as many neurons of this class support lengthy axon projections. Most pyramidal cells send their axon out of the cortical region to synapse. The stellate cells are the principal intrinsic neurons. Two subtypes have been observed in cytoarchitectural studies of visual cortex. Spiny stellate cells are excitatory, whereas the aspinous stellate cells are principally inhibitory local circuit neurons. Many of these inhibitory intrinsic neurons use γ-aminobutyric acid (GABA) as a synaptic transmitter. Fusiform cells populate lower cortical layers, and a variety of other neuronal cell types are found. Glial cells are present throughout, providing myelin, structural, and metabolic support.

The six layers can be distinguished in cell-stained cross section (Fig. 8-4). The outer molecular layer is cell-poor and composed mainly of neuropil (nerve cell processes and glia). Many fibers in layer I are tangentially oriented. Layer II, the external granular cell layer, is a composition of mixed cell types. Layers III and V are dominated by the pyramidal cells. The corticospinal tract originates from the giant pyramidal cells of Betz in layer V of the primary motor cortex. Layer IV, the internal granular cell layer, is a dense layer of stellate cells, best developed in sensory cortex. Specific thalamic afferents terminate here. Layer VI is known as the multiform layer.

Cell stains define the principal neuronal types and cortical layers, but other methods are required to analyze the connections of cortical neurons. The Golgi stain is an excellent technique for studying neuronal processes (Fig. 8-5). A capricious silver stain, it produces a beautiful and complete impregnation of a small subset of nerve cells, leaving many of the background cells unstained. It is thus possible to trace neuronal processes and regional connections, to appreciate the full dendritic arbor and even the spines on which synaptic contacts occur. Though only a small percentage of cells are stained, one can begin to visualize some of the network relationships of cortical nerve cells.

Evidence is overwhelming that the basic organizational unit of the neocortex is its vertical column. Comparative studies show that the column is the building block of large cortical structures. During development, neurons migrate to their adult positions in the cortex vertically, along radial guide paths. As the cortex is populated, neurites follow the same tissue planes in seeking synaptic contacts. The apical dendrite of pyramidal neurons, its logical "backbone," is oriented vertically within the column. Cortical nerve cells are thus richly interconnected along their vertical axis; sparsely so horizontally. Physiologic recording from sensory cortex has established that cells along a vertical axis share physiologic properties with regard to their receptive field (that part of sensory space in which a stimulus influences the firing of a cell).

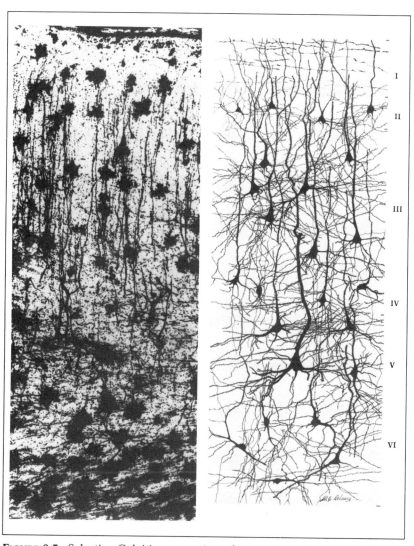

FIGURE 8-5. Selective Golgi impregnation of cortex from the same region shown in Figure 8-4. On right is a camera lucida drawing of some of the cortical neurons which took the stain. (Reprinted by permission from J.L. Conel, *The Post Natal Development of the Cerebral Cortex.* Cambridge, Mass.: Harvard University Press, 1959, Vol. 6.)

Studies of physiology have also taught us about regional specializations of the cerebral cortex. In the 1950s Penfield studied the human cortex in patients having surgery for epilepsy. It was often necessary to partially wake the patient intraoperatively to map out functional

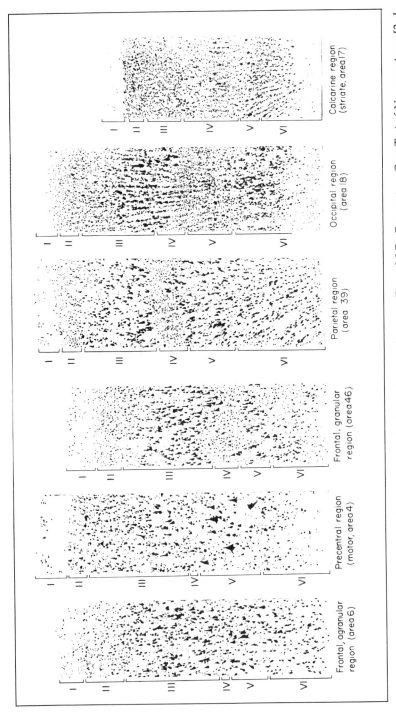

FIGURE 8-6. The cytoarchitectural differences in six distinct cortical areas. (From M.B. Carpenter, *Core Text of Neuroanatomy* [3rd ed.]. P. 350, © 1986, the Williams & Wilkins Co., Baltimore.)

anatomy, in order to avoid surgery on areas vital for language or motor control. Penfield found areas in which stimulation evoked a specific sensation or a motor response. Within the somatosensory cortex of the postcentral gyrus and primary motor cortex (precentral), studies showed a precisely ordered map of the body wall onto the cortical surface (a *somatotopic* projection). Similar ordered mappings have been observed in animal physiology on primary visual cortex and auditory cortex (retinotopic and tonotopic projections). Regional differences in cytoarchitecture correspond to the observed functional specializations (Fig. 8-6). Sensory cortex has a well-developed internal granular cell layer (layer IV). Motor and premotor cortex contain abundant pyramidal cells. Association cortex contains a more even mix, with many stellate cells in the upper layers. Brodmann developed criteria for evaluation of a cortex according to its structural detail. He was able to sort the cerebral cortex into 47 distinct cytoarchitectonic fields (Fig. 8-7). His map has been a guide for all subsequent studies of cortical specializations.

Just as there are regional specializations in cortical function and regional differences in cytoarchitecture, there are also important differences in connectivity. Areas of cortex receive different patterns of extrinsic connections. Primary visual cortex (area 17), for example, receives inputs from the lateral geniculate body, a thalamic nucleus of the visual system. Somatosensory cortex (areas 1, 2, and 3) receives thalamic afferents from the ventral posterolateral (VPL) and ventral posteromedial (VPM) nuclei concerning pain, touch localization, and joint position sense. This cortex cannot conceivably ponder visual issues, as it lacks the relevant afferent information. To a large degree, afferent connections *determine* functional specialization. This observation raises a broader question about cortical organization: How is function related to cytoarchitecture, and to what degree are function and cytoarchitecture determined by the pattern of cortical connections (inputs and outputs)? A reasonable hypothesis holds that cortex begins embryonic life as somewhat equipotential. As connections are made and redundant cellular elements are lost in late prenatal, early postnatal development, cortex becomes anatomically specialized and functionally dedicated. Studies by Hubel and Wiesel suggest that early experience and use of cortical structures during a critical period of development determine the final pattern of synaptic connections.

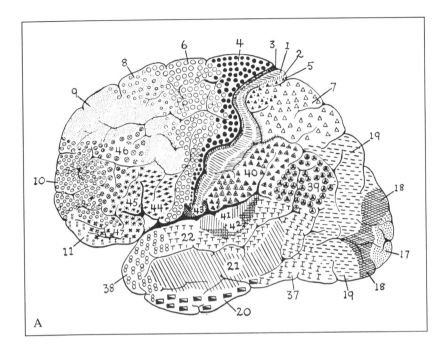

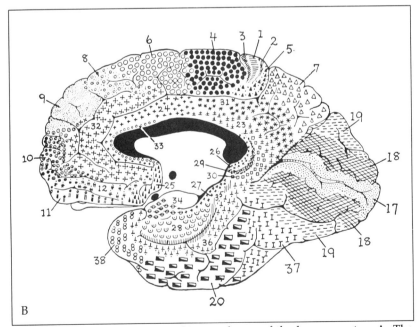

FIGURE 8-7. Brodmann's cytoarchitectural map of the human cortex. A. The convexity. B. The medial surface. Forty-seven different cytoarchitectonic fields can be distinguished. (From M.B. Carpenter, *Core Text of Neuroanatomy* [3rd ed.]. P. 355, © 1986, the Williams & Wilkins Co., Baltimore.)

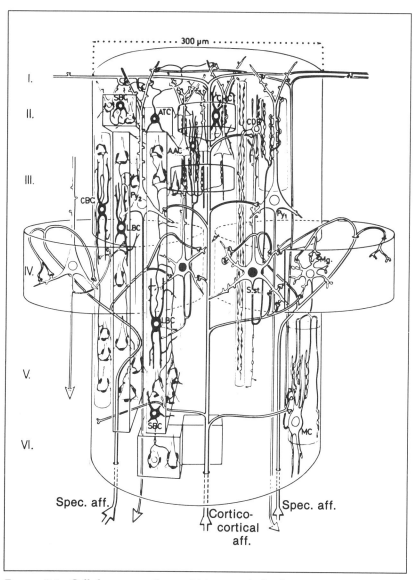

FIGURE 8-8. Cellular connections within a cortical column, as conceptualized by Szentagothai. Excitatory cells are outlined, while inhibitory cells are shown in black. The excitatory connections of a spiny stellate cell are shown on the right. Pyramidal cell (Py₂, *on left*) operates under the filter of large basket cells (LBC), chandelier cells (CHC), and axoaxonic cells (AAC). The two flat cylinders in lamina IV correspond to the termination territory of a specific afferent. SBC = small basket cell; S.st. = spiny stellate cell; MC = Martinotti cell; Mg. = microgliform interneurons; ATC = axonal tufted cells; CBC = inhibitory columnar basket cells; CDB = *cellules a double bouquet*. (From F.O. Schmitt and F.G. Worden [eds.], *The Neurosciences, Fourth Study Program*. Cambridge, Mass.: MIT Press, 1980, p. 408, with permission.)

The Cortical Column

A closer look at the cortical column reveals the workings of this basic unit of information processing. The cortex can be imagined as a modular design, a large array of cortical columns. The vertical column is the "microchip" of the neocortex, and the cortical mantle has an abundance of parallel processors. Figure 8-8 shows the conceptualization of the Hungarian neuroanatomist Szentagothai, depicting cellular connections within a cortical column. *Intrinsic connections* provide the resident intelligence of the cortical microcircuit. The spines on apical dendrites of pyramidal cells integrate incoming information; a precise correlation set of synaptic events will elicit depolarization of the pyramidal cell. *Extrinsic connections* determine the input-output relations of the column. Specific thalamic afferents arrive in layer IV; afferents from brainstem and nonspecific thalamic nuclei are present in all layers. Corticocortical connections exit from layer III; subcortical projections like the corticospinal tract originate in layers V and VI (Fig. 8-9).

There are also important lateral connections with adjacent cortical columns. In the visual cortex, Hubel and Wiesel have shown that cortical columns influence processing in neighboring columns. The optimal stimulus (receptive field) for stellate cells in layer IVc of visual cortex is a contrasting annulus of center and opposite surround. More complex visual perceptions can be built by composition of these elements. Surround inhibition is thought to be a general design feature of cortical systems. This design heightens contrast in sensory processing.

Regional Specializations

Each of the two cerebral hemispheres has regions dedicated to motor function and sensory processing. In the frontal lobe, primary motor cortex (Brodmann's area 4) occupies the precentral gyrus. The adjacent cortical regions, including the frontal eye fields and supplementary motor area, are motor association areas. Primary visual cortex lines the calcarine fissure in the medial occipital lobe, surrounded by

---

FIGURE 8-9. Simplified wiring diagram of the cortex. Large pyramidal cells (*white*) in layers III and V receive multiple synaptic contacts from the stellate cell (*stippled*) in layer IV. Inhibitory basket cell (*in black*) is directed to neighboring cortical neurons. This pattern of circuitry underlies surround inhibition (after Szentagothai, 1969). (From E.R. Kandel and J.H. Schwartz, *Principles of Neural Science* [2nd ed.]. New York: Elsevier, 1985, p. 637, with permission.)

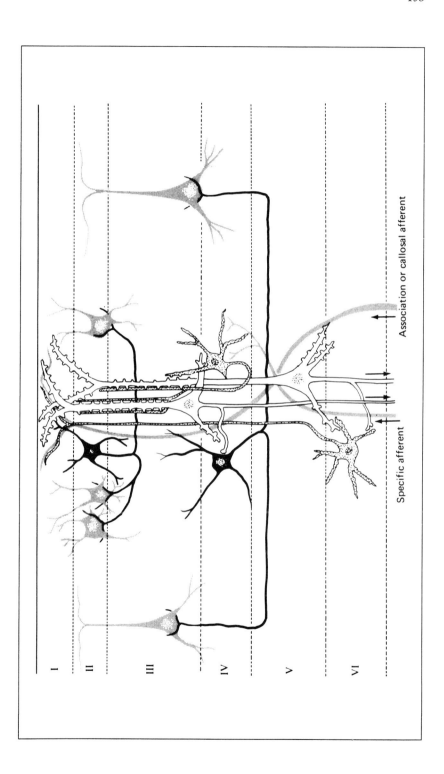

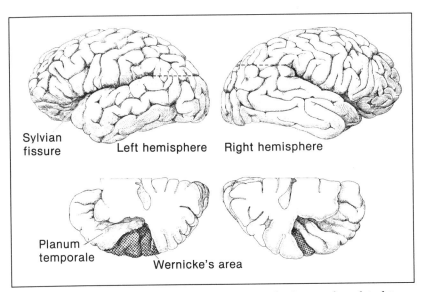

Sylvian fissure   Left hemisphere   Right hemisphere

Planum temporale   Wernicke's area

FIGURE 8-10. Anatomic asymmetry in the human brain may be related to the functional specialization of the hemispheres. The sylvian fissure, which defines the upper margin of the temporal lobe, rises more steeply in the right hemisphere. Within the planum temporale, exposed when the sylvian fissure is opened, another asymmetry is observed. The posterior part is usually much larger on the left side. (From N. Geschwind, Specializations of the human brain. *Scientific American*, September 1979, p. 115, with permission.)

visual association areas. Auditory cortex is in the temporal lobe, along the transverse gyrus of Heschl. The parietal lobe on either side contains the postcentral gyrus, a primary sensory cortex for somatosensory processing. Somatosensory association cortex includes the superior parietal lobule; the inferior parietal lobule is a higher-order, multimodal association cortex. These regions of the parietal lobe provide an internal map of the contralateral body wall and its relation to extrapersonal space.

The corpus callosum is a great white matter commissure which coordinates the activities of homologous regions of the two hemispheres. But the two cerebral hemispheres are not identical mirror-image structures. There are well-described anatomic asymmetries and interhemispheric specializations. Geschwind and Levitsky have shown that the sylvian fissure is longer and more horizontal on the left (Fig. 8-10). Detailed cytoarchitectural studies by Galaburda on the superior temporal gyrus show that area Tpt, a part of the auditory association cortex specialized for language, is 7 times greater in size on the left for most individuals. Gross asymmetries of cortical regions are present in the third trimester of human fetal development, and are

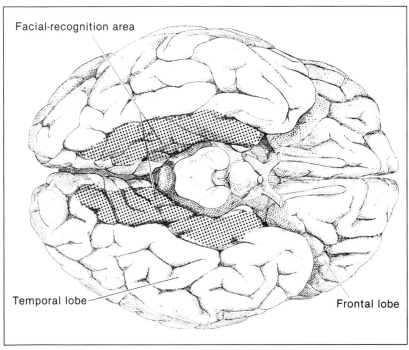

Facial-recognition area

Temporal lobe

Frontal lobe

FIGURE 8-11. Area on the underside of the occipitotemporal region on both sides is essential to the task of face recognition. A bilateral lesion in this area results in prosopagnosia (see text). (From N. Geschwind, Specialization of the human brain. *Scientific American*, September 1979, p. 114, with permission.)

also reflected in examination of the early fossil record. Skulls of Neanderthal man, dated 30,000 to 50,000 years, and Peking man (300,000 years old) show asymmetries of the planum temporale, as manifest on the inner table of the skull. For 97 percent of the human population the left cerebral hemisphere contains regions specialized for language. While the left hemisphere is dominant for language, the right hemisphere is far from dormant. It is specialized for analysis of visuospatial relations, aspects of directed attention, and emotional expression.

Much of what we understand about the specialized role of cortical areas comes from the study of patients with brain injury and stroke. It is difficult to study such human functions in any animal model. Some caution is required in interpreting lesion studies. As an example, we consider the special case of prosopagnosia. Recognition of faces is a particularly developed facility of the human central nervous system (CNS). It is a skill present in early life. An infant can recognize a human face from birth, and can recognize his or her mother from several weeks. Adults can pick out an acquaintance from a sea of faces, or from a photograph taken at some remote point in time. Caricature is

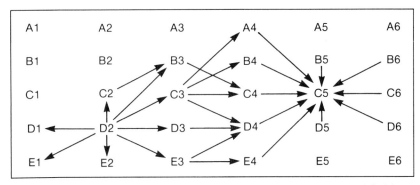

FIGURE 8-12. Information processing in a cortical network. Cortical fields A1 through E6 are linked via a network of corticocortical connections. Information processing occurs in this fashion through a wealth of divergent and convergent connections. This architecture fosters analysis by feature extraction, pattern recognition, and thereby associative thought. When centers with shared function are widely distributed in different regions, the arrangement is referred to as a distributed network.

perhaps the epitome of such talent: a cartoon figure which may be a poor likeness stands for a specific person in our mind's eye. A bilateral lesion on the underside of the occipital lobe produces prosopagnosia—the inability to recognize faces (Fig. 8-11). The patient cannot associate the name with a face, and may fail to recognize members of his or her own family. Voice recognition in such patients is unimpaired. What does the peculiar deficit associated with this lesion tell us about the organization of the brain? We *cannot* infer that the skill for face recognition resides there. Rather we learn that data processing essential for the task is done by this cortical region and its connections.

In addition to the corpus callosum, which links regions of the two hemispheres, there is a vast network of intrahemispheric corticocortical connections. As a general principle, all corticocortical connections are routed through association cortex. This routing is somewhat indirect, but allows an orderly flow of information. A single exception is the interconnection of primary motor and primary somatosensory cortex across the central sulcus: homunculus to homunculus. Within a cortical field, not all columns enjoy the same remote connections. A subset (a "macrocolumn") will have specific connections with selected subsets of other cortical fields. When remote cortical areas cooperate on a processing task, this arrangement is known as a distributed network (Fig. 8-12). Divergent and convergent connections allow us to form particular associations, and to handle information by feature extraction. No one has derived a computational theory about how this might be done, but the ability to form symbolic associations and construct associations lists has been the basis for some computer simulations of human intelligence.

DISORDERS OF CORTICAL FUNCTION

We assess the function of cerebral cortex at the bedside using the mental status examination, an important tool in neurologic diagnosis. Further help is available from the laboratory in the form of the electroencephalogram (EEG) and standardized neuropsychologic tests. The mental status examination always includes a statement on the patient's sensorium: alertness, orientation. Assessment proceeds to the patient's mood and the *quality of attention.* Fund of knowledge is checked with a few general questions, as knowledge is a general property of mental state. Speech and language testing look at the competence of left hemisphere language areas. Memory is tested by requesting that the patient remember a few details. The information is retrieved after an interval of several minutes of doing something else (distraction). Visuospatial skills of the right parietal lobe are examined, including the ability to reproduce drawings (constructional ability). Insight and judgment are thought to reside in the frontal lobe. Capacity for abstract thought is sometimes examined with similarities and proverb interpretations.

Disorders of cortical function may be restricted (focal) in nature. More general global or multifocal abnormalities are also seen. The distinction is a useful one, even though many global disorders have particular salient features. Dementia and delirium are examples of more widespread disorders of cortical function.

Dementia

Persistent loss of mental function (dementia) is a common problem among the elderly. Studies suggest that 10 to 15 percent of persons over 65 meet formal diagnostic criteria. A diagnosis of dementia requires sustained loss of intellectual function (memory, language, abstract thought, visuospatial ability, social skill) in the absence of a clouded sensorium. The diagnosis cannot be confirmed in a sleepy or inattentive patient. Common causes of a dementia syndrome are listed in Table 8-1. Workup is done in an attempt to identify a reversible cause of mental decline.

About half the patients have Alzheimer's disease, a degenerative disorder of the cortex and forebrain. Alzheimer's disease is a slowly progressive dementia, age-related with onset in mid- to late adult life. Clinically, patients display rapid decay of verbal and nonverbal memory. Visuospatial ability is often impaired early. Speech is typically vacuous and circumlocutory, with some naming errors. Personality and social behavior may be relatively preserved at an early stage. The clinical picture is not specific, and pathologic studies show a 10 to 15 percent error rate in clinical diagnosis.

TABLE 8-1. Common Causes of a Dementia Syndrome

Cause	Percent
Degenerative	
Alzheimer's disease	55.0
Pick's disease	0.3
Parkinson's disease	1.2
Progressive supranuclear palsy	0.9
Huntington's disease	0.9
Other	1.0
Vascular	
Multi-infarct dementia	10.0
Mixed (Alzheimer's with infarcts)	4.0
Toxic, metabolic, nutritional	
Chronic Korsakoff syndrome	4.0
Hypothyroidism	0.2
Chronic hepatocerebral degeneration	0.3
Dialysis dementia	0.5
Vitamin B_{12} deficiency	0.2
Other metabolic	0.5
Drug effects	1.5
Structural	
Intracranial tumor ($\pm$ radiation)	1.5
Head trauma	1.0
Normal-pressure hydrocephalus	2.0
Chronic infectious or inflammatory	
Neurosyphilis	0.1
Acquired immunodeficiency syndrome dementia	?
Creutzfeldt-Jakob disease	0.3
Pseudodementia (depression, etc.)	7.0

Source: Data derived by averaging various clinical series (meta-analysis), including those of Wells (Chronic brain disease: An overview. *Am. J. Psych.* 135 : 1–12, 1978) and Smith (The investigation of dementia: Results in 200 consecutive admissions. Lancet 1 : 824–827, 1981).

Postmortem studies show gross atrophy of the cerebral cortex, most pronounced in association areas. Senile plaques and neurofibrillary tangles are evident in microscopic examination of the cortex and hippocampus (Fig. 8-13). The plaque count (number of senile plaques per high-power field) is correlated with the clinical severity of the dementia. Plaques and tangles contain paired helical filaments, the residual protein skeleton of nerve cells that have undergone degeneration. There is marked cell loss in the septal nucleus and basal nucleus of Meynert, the source of cholinergic projections to the hippocampus and neocortex.

Another pathologic feature of Alzheimer's disease is the deposition of β-pleated protein (amyloid) in senile plaques and cerebral blood vessels. Amyloid proteins in the CNS have been proposed as a molec-

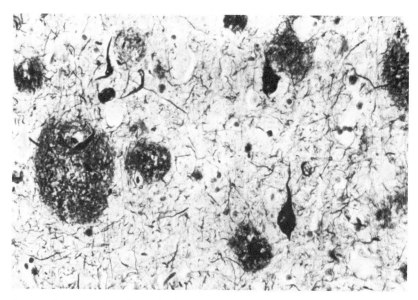

FIGURE 8-13. Section through the cortex stained with Bielschowsky's silver stain shows senile plaques (the round blobs) and neurons stuffed with neurofibrillary tangles. These lesions are the cytoskeletal markers characteristic of Alzheimer's disease.

ular marker for Alzheimer's disease. Some cases of Alzheimer's disease, perhaps 10 percent or more, appear to be genetically determined. Linkage studies in a few families have identified a defect on chromosome 21. This finding is of particular interest as the β-amyloid precursor gene is on chromosome 21. Patients with trisomy 21 (Down's syndrome) often have a form of premature Alzheimer's disease. However, there is presently no evidence for overproduction of amyloid precursor proteins in other forms of Alzheimer's. Pruisner and co-workers propose that proteinaceous infectious particles (prions) are the cause of the histologic changes in Alzheimer's disease. The cause of the disease remains a topic of active interest and controversy.

Aphasia

The term *aphasia* refers to an acquired disorder of language, due to brain injury or disease. It does not include slurred speech (dysarthria) or mutism; the aphasic patient produces linguistically abnormal speech. Several different syndromes are recognized. We consider three basic aphasia types in more detail.

In the 1860s Paul Broca reported the curious case of a patient named LeBorgne. After suffering a stroke, LeBorgne had a right hemiparesis and a language abnormality. He had severely restricted speech output; speech was limited to a single word—*tan*. Nonetheless, he understood spoken language well, and was able to communicate using gestures. In 1861 he died and an autopsy was done, demonstrating injury to a region of the left frontal lobe, including area 44, a region now known as Broca's area. Subsequently, Broca examined a few patients with stroke involving the homologous region on the right who did not have aphasia. He postulated that this part of the left hemisphere, area 44 in the frontal operculum, was an important center for language output.

We now recognize a syndrome characterized by poor speech output, abnormal rhythm and prosody (the musical quality of speech), and severely limited phrase length. Patients with Broca's aphasia have telegraphic speech: their word-strings rarely exceed three to four words in length. They generally lack the short, functionally important words that indicate syntactic structure (words like *if, and, but, by, for*). They have a deficit in the organization of speech output and aspects of grammar. Studies by Mohr and co-workers have shown that area 44 is the core area of damage in patients with Broca's aphasia. Aphasia is not invariably present when small lesions are restricted to area 44; aphasia is seemingly more common with larger strokes.

In 1874 Karl Wernicke discovered a second speech area in the left hemisphere. His patient had a stroke involving the superior temporal gyrus, the auditory association cortex just behind areas 41 and 42. The principal language areas in the left hemisphere are illustrated in Figure 8-14. Wernicke's area includes those parts of the superior temporal gyrus where cytoarchitectural specializations for language in the left hemisphere have been demonstrated. It presumably functions to decode an incoming utterance into phonetic components, words, and ultimately language. The syndrome described by Wernicke is contrasted with Broca's aphasia in Table 8-2. It is a quite different disorder of language. The patient's spontaneous speech is fully fluent, often rather rambling, and may contain greater than the normal density of words. It also contains phonetic and literal substitutions (paraphasic errors) and some nonsense words, and sounds rather confused. Comprehension of spoken language is grossly impaired, and the patient may be altogether unaware that he is not making sense.

Wernicke's area is connected to Broca's area by a white matter tract, the arcuate fasciculus (see Fig. 8-14), which runs deep through the sylvian region. A third speech area is found in the inferior parietal lobule of the left hemisphere, the angular gyrus area. This region is thought to contain the semantic field or dictionary, where words are paired with their associations. Comprehension of spoken language involves processing in the primary auditory cortex (areas 41, 42), decoding of linguistic components of the utterance in Wernicke's area,

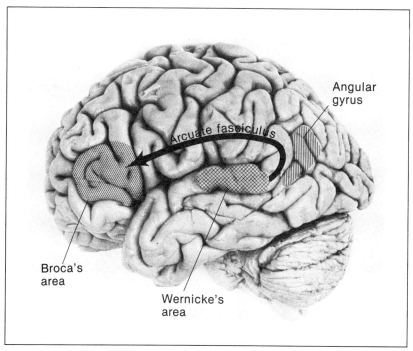

FIGURE 8-14. Language areas of the left hemisphere: Broca's area in the left frontal operculum mediates aspects of speech production. Wernicke's area in the superior temporal gyrus is essential for comprehension. They are joined by a white matter tract, the arcuate fasciculus. A lesion anywhere along this pathway interferes with repetition of spoken language. The angular gyrus area is a semantic field, in which words are matched with their meaning. (Adapted from N. Geschwind, Specialization of the human brain. *Scientific American,* 1979, p. 116, with permission.)

and ultimately semantic analysis in the angular gyrus. Repetition of speech uses a different anatomy. The spoken phrase is again parsed in Wernicke's area, but is then fed forward along the arcuate fasciculus from Wernicke's to Broca's area. Motor speech instructions are assembled in Broca's area, and sent to the motor cortex on either side. These instructions are then implemented by the cortical segment representing the mouth, pharynx, and larynx. Based on the anatomy, one might predict a third aphasia syndrome due to interruption of the arcuate fasciculus. Such patients would have fluent, paraphasic speech, good comprehension, but a total inability to repeat a spoken phrase. Such a syndrome is observed, and is known as *conduction aphasia* (see Table 8-2). Aphasic disorders are occasionally seen with left hemisphere lesions outside the perisylvian area. In such cases repetition is preserved, a useful discriminating feature.

TABLE 8-2. Characteristics of Principal Aphasic Disorders

	Broca's Aphasia	Wernicke's Syndrome	Conduction Aphasia
Spontaneous speech	Nonfluent	Fluent, paraphasic	Fluent, paraphasic
Comprehension	Full	Nil	Good
Repetition	Poor	Absent	Absent
Right-sided paralysis	Always present	Slight or none	Slight or none

The Nondominant Parietal Lobe Syndrome

A profound disturbance of perception and behavior often accompanies lesions of the parietal lobe, lesions which may be unassociated with a language or motor deficit. The parietal lobe takes its name from the lateral wall of the hemisphere which it occupies. In a larger sense, the parietal lobe is concerned with relations of the body wall to extrapersonal space.

Mountcastle has emphasized the role of the parietal lobe in the integration of sensory stimuli relative to contralateral exploratory behavior. His primates with parietal lesions displayed a paucity of arm movements into contralateral space. When movements were elicited, the animals made errors in the direction and depth of their reaching behavior. In recording from the parietal lobe of normal waking monkeys, he demonstrated cells in area 7 of the inferior parietal lobule concerned with visual fixation, visual tracking, and visually evoked motor behavior. Human patients with lesions in this region display a reduction in exploratory movements on the opposite side, even when limb strength is full.

The deficits observed with parietal lobe lesions of man can be considered in two parts. The first consists of deficits contralateral to the side of the lesion, primarily deficits in sensory integration. Mountcastle calls this "the purely contralateral syndrome." Deficits include astereognosis, impaired graphesthesia, poor two-point discrimination, and misreaching into contralateral visual space. In contrast, the "bilateral syndrome" is a gross deficit in the patient's perception and behavior, specifically related to the nondominant hemisphere. Patients with right parietal lesions have a profound disturbance of visuospatial skills. They may, for example, be unable to interpret maps, give directions, or describe or draw the floor plan of their house. Their attempts at copying constructions are often grossly deranged with regard to external design (constructional apraxia). They may specifi-

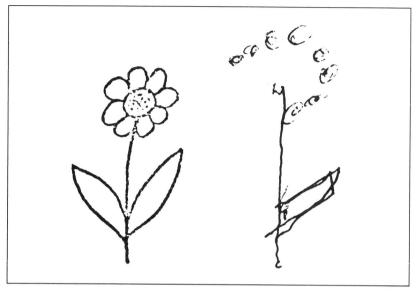

FIGURE 8-15. An example of hemispatial neglect. Patient with a right parietal lesion omits the left half of the figure he is attempting to copy (*on left*). (From K. Heilman and E. Valenstein, *Clinical Neuropsychology* [2nd ed.]. New York: Oxford University Press, 1985, p. 246, with permission.)

cally omit the left half of copied figures (Fig. 8-15). This omission is associated with an underlying behavioral neglect of the left body and left sensory space, which may be profound. Patients have been known not to recognize a paretic left arm as their own, or to complain that another patient has gotten into bed with them. This abnormal body image and neglect may include anosognosia: denial of the patient's illness and deficits.

Disconnection Syndromes

We have reviewed several neurologic disorders which occur as a result of lesions in focal areas essential to a particular task, such as Broca's aphasia, constructional apraxia, and prosopagnosia. Conduction aphasia is unique among the syndromes described, in that the dysfunction is due solely to interruption of a white matter tract. No cortical centers are injured; only the connection between Broca's and Wernicke's area is disabled. Conduction aphasia is an example of a disconnection syndrome: a neurologic deficit due to interruption of white matter connections between cortical areas. Disconnection syndromes are important because they illustrate the functional reliance of neocortex on

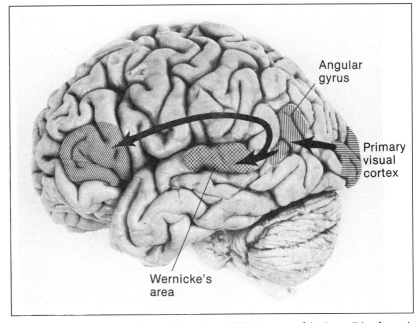

FIGURE 8-16. Anatomy for reading aloud. Written word is "seen" in the primary visual area of the occipital lobe, and relayed forward to the angular gyrus. There the written form of the word is associated with its meaning. With the help of Wernicke's area, the words are passed forward to articulate speech.

appropriate extrinsic connections. They also underscore the need to think of the forebrain as a composition, or network, of specialized areas, and not as an organ with uniform distribution function (like the lung or the kidney). When a complex performance fails in a patient with neurologic disease, we must always inquire, What is the normal anatomy for that task?

A particular example is the syndrome of alexia without agraphia, or "pure word blindness." This syndrome was first described by Dejerine in 1894. His patient, a highly educated man with some musical talent, sustained a stroke in the left occipital lobe. This left him with no paralysis or sensory loss, but a right homonymous hemianopia (inability to see in the right visual field). The patient had good vision for the left half of space, and no neglect syndrome, so he was able to compensate for his loss by making an extra effort to look around. As he convalesced from his stroke, the patient became aware of a rather curious disorder of written language. The patient spoke clearly and understood spoken language. He was, however, totally unable to read. He could write to dictation, but was unable minutes later to read

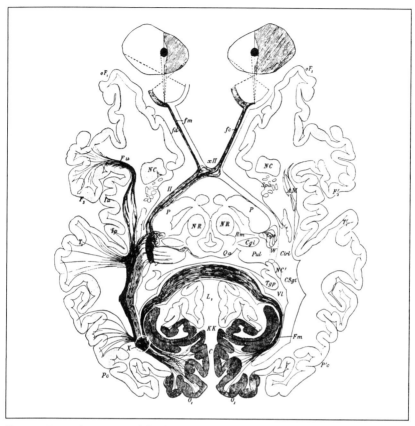

FIGURE 8-17. Anatomy of the lesion in Dejerine's patient. Horizontal section through the "zone of language" in the sylvian fossa. The lesion in the left occipitotemporal region is marked with an X. This lesion destroys the optic radiations in the left occipital lobe, and the posterior fifth of the corpus callosum. Information in the right visual cortex (from the good field of vision) cannot reach the left hemisphere language areas.

what he himself had written. This deficit included printed text, script, and also the inability to read music. It was a frustrating and persistent disability.

The anatomy for reading aloud is reviewed in Figure 8-16. Text is "seen" in area 17, the primary visual cortex. The visual association cortex from the occipital lobe communicates with the angular gyrus area, where the words are associated with their meaning. Information of a linguistic nature is passed anteriorly through Wernicke's area and the arcuate fasciculus to Broca's area for speech production. A dominant-hemisphere, posterior cerebral artery territory infarct is illustrated in the horizontal schematic in Figure 8-17. The stroke involves the left occipital lobe and the posterior fifth of the corpus callosum. The left occipital lobe lacks function, resulting in a right homonymous hemianopia. The right occipital lobe is preserved. In order to read, information from the right visual association cortex would need to be transferred to left hemisphere language areas. The callosal infarct disconnects these cortical areas, so that the angular gyrus has no access to the visual image of the text.

The term *apraxia* is sometimes seen in the literature on cortical function. Apraxia denotes an inability to carry out a motor act to command, despite preservation of motor and sensory function, comprehension, and full cooperation. The term has been used quite liberally in contemporary neurology (gait apraxia, oculomotor apraxia, dressing apraxia). The most characteristic and pure apraxia is the inability of some aphasic patients to protrude the tongue or to use the muscles of the face or left arm to perform a familiar act on command. The patient may fail when asked, "Show how you would blow out a match," or "Show how you would comb your hair." Often these learned movements can be elicited by giving the patient the appropriate object to use, thus demonstrating that there is no deficit in the motor skill. In this case, interruption of callosal pathways in the anterior left hemisphere limits transfer of the command instructions to the intact right hemisphere for execution. Seeing the lighted match, the right hemisphere may cue the appropriate movement (pursing the lips and blowing air to extinguish the flame). In general terms, a disconnection syndrome is a deficit in which cortical regions fail to work together because of an interruption of their connections. The functional capabilities of the cortex are limited by a disorder of extrinsic connections.

LIMBIC SYSTEM

The limbic system is that part of the forebrain concerned with emotions. Neocortical structures of the cerebrum handle sensory analysis, language, computation, and associative thought—rational functions of human intelligence. Unlike a computer, however, humans possess moods, animal drives, and species-typical emotional behaviors, which can be quite irrational at times. The hypothalamus and autonomic nervous system are generally thought of as a "visceral brain." These deep structures get no direct neocortical input about our external environment. Since our behavioral repertoire is complex, we need a cortical structure to provide oversight. The limbic system, a network of telencephalic structures and their connections, manages this interface. Diseases of the limbic system often produce complex disturbances in emotion, motivation, and memory.

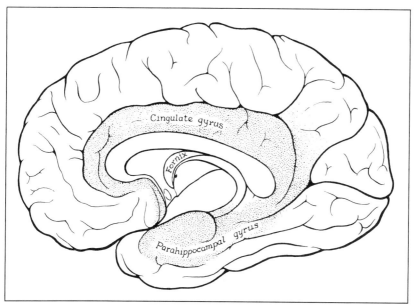

FIGURE 8-18. The limbic lobe of Broca: a ring of structures in the medial wall of the cerebral hemisphere. Hippocampus, cingulate gyrus, septal area, and amygdala are included. (From M.B. Carpenter, *Core Text of Neuroanatomy* [3rd ed.]. P. 346. © 1986, the Williams & Wilkins Co., Baltimore).

The term *limbic lobe,* first used by Paul Broca in the nineteenth century, refers to a ring of cortical structures in the mesial wall of the cerebral hemisphere (Fig. 8-18). Generally included are the hippocampus and parahippocampal gyrus, the cingulate gyrus, the subcallosal gyrus, and the septal area. The amygdala, a part of the basal ganglia, is usually thrown in for good measure. These are phylogenetically older, non-neocortical structures. The term *limbic system,* by contrast, is more inclusive, referring to a network of associated structures, a functional grouping. The limbic system includes the hypothalamus, the medial dorsal, central medial, and anterior thalamic nuclei, the habenula, and the tegmental area of the midbrain. It also encompasses parts of the frontal lobe and the insular cortex. These structures are concerned with aspects of emotional state and behavior. Anatomy texts include the limbic system together with the olfactory system, as they share a common origin. The olfactory tracts enjoy direct access to structures of the limbic lobe. There has been substantial divergence of function in higher animals, best illustrated in the brains of whales and dolphins. These animals enjoy considerable telencephalic development, and have a large limbic lobe, but they totally lack olfaction. As limbic structures have expanded during primate evolution, olfaction

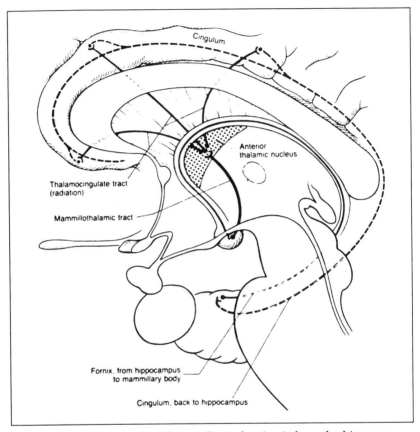

FIGURE 8-19. Sulcal circuit of Papez: Trace the circuit from the hippocampus, via the fornix, to the mammillary nucleus of the hypothalamus. The mammillothalamic tract leads to the anterior thalamic nuclei. From there, projections lead to the cingulate gyrus, and along the cingulum to the parahippocampal gyrus. (Reprinted by permission from Duus, P.: *Topical Diagnosis in Neurology*, Thieme Medical Publishers, New York, 1983.)

has diminished in importance. The sense of smell is related to eating and sexual behavior to some degree, even among primates, but the primary function of the limbic system is not olfactory processing.

The principal pathway which interconnects limbic structures is the sulcal circuit of Papez (Fig. 8-19). This circuit forms a loop (a reentrant pathway) in each hemisphere, joined at the hippocampal commissure, where there is a small amount of cross talk. To trace the pathway, begin at the fornix bundle. This hippocampal efferent pathway contains 1.2 million axons, and is comparable in size to the optic nerve. It runs under the corpus callosum, and splits at the anterior

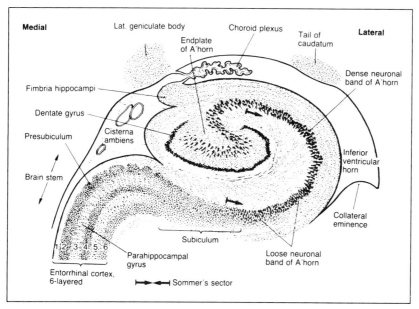

Medial Lat. geniculate body Choroid plexus Tail of **Lateral**
caudatum

Endplate
of A'horn

Dense neuronal
band of A'horn

Fimbria hippocampi

Dentate gyrus

Presubiculum Cisterna
ambiens

Inferior
ventricular
horn

Brain stem

Collateral
eminence

1 2 3 4 5 6 Subiculum

Parahippocampal Loose neuronal
gyrus band of A'horn

Entorrhinal cortex,
6-layered Sommer's sector

FIGURE 8-20. The hippocampal formation: Dorsal to the hippocampal fissure lies the dentate gyrus and Ammon's horn (A'horn). The cells of Sommer's sector (*marked by arrows*) are vulnerable to ischemia. (Reprinted by permission from Duus, P.: *Topical Diagnosis in Neurology*, Thieme Medical Publishers, New York, 1983.)

commisure, to terminate in the septal area and mammillary nucleus of the hypothalamus. The mamillothalamic tract connects the mammillary nucleus with the limbic thalamus, which in turn projects to the cingulate gyrus. The cingulum bundle connects through to the parahippocampal gyrus, which is the principal source of hippocampal afferents. Papez thought that this reverberating circuit might be important in aspects of limbic system processing, particularly as a register for emotional state.

Hippocampus

The hippocampal formation includes the dentate gyrus and the horn of Ammon, structures dorsal to the hippocampal fissure (Fig. 8-20). Across the fissure lies the transitional cortex of the parahippocampal gyrus and the subiculum. The hippocampus is a well-studied structure, as it is possible to do detailed physiologic studies on an in vitro preparation of hippocampal slice. The microcircuit anatomy and

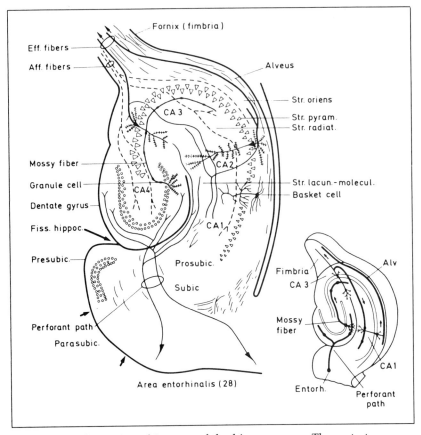

FIGURE 8-21. Synaptic architecture of the hippocampus. Three strata, or layers, are seen. Principal (pyramidal) cell layer is inverted. Axons of CA1 and subiculum pyramidal cells collect in the alveus and exit via the fornix. Inset shows the trisynaptic circuit from the entorhinal area of the parahippocampal gyrus to the dentate gyrus, to CA3 pyramidal cells, to CA1 pyramidal cells. (From A. Brodal, *Neurological Anatomy* [3rd ed.]. New York: Oxford University Press, 1981, p. 675, with permission.)

neurotransmitter connections are consequently quite well known, yet we still have a fairly limited idea about their function.

The three-layered cortical structure is detailed in Figure 8-21. Hippocampal cortex is inside out, in the sense that the white matter efferents are on the surface. The pyramidal cell is the principal cell type; its apical dendrites are oriented downward (upside down). The pyramidal cell layer extends across the hippocampal fissure into the subiculum. Outgoing axons of subiculum and CA1 pyramidal cells collect as the alveus to form the fimbria, the root of the fornix bundle. The fornix is the principal efferent pathway of the hippocampus.

Afferents come from the entorhinal area of the parahippocampal gyrus, via the perforant pathway. Cholinergic afferents derive from the septal area. The perforant path (so named because it perforates the hippocampal fissure) terminates in the distal fields (CA3, CA4, and the dentate gyrus). A cascade of (Shaeffer) axon collaterals from pyramidal cells leads back outward along the spiral. A trisynaptic circuit within the hippocampal formation is often described. The perforant path neurons of the entorhinal area terminate in the dentate gyrus in an excitatory synapse. Dentate granule cells send axons to the large pyramidal cells of CA3. CA3 pyramidal cell axons are excitatory onto pyramidal cells of CA2 CA1. CA1 pyramidal cells send their axons out via the fimbria-fornix pathway, with a recurrent collateral back to the entorhinal area.

Studies suggest that the hippocampus marks events for storage in memory. Not all experiences are of equivalent value, and we don't remember all things equally well. The hippocampus provides a marker of the *emotional valence* of events, so that they may be selectively etched in our memory. A physiologic specialization within hippocampal circuits may assist in this task. At some synapses, the strength of transmission increases with repetitive use. When this effect persists for more than a few minutes, it is called *long-term potentiation* (LTP). LTP has been demonstrated at excitatory synapses onto the principal neurons of the hippocampus. A cooperative effect, or pairing of synaptic inputs, is necessary. Simultaneous activity of convergent inputs onto CA3 or CA1 pyramidal cells can condition the excitatory synapse, so as to enhance its subsequent effectiveness. Calcium influx at the open (or unblocked) N-methyl-*d*-aspartate (NMDA) receptor may be the specific trigger for synaptic modification. This phenomenon may be important in the physiology of memory consolidation through the hippocampal circuit.

Amnesia is the inability to remember new information. Such a deficit is often associated with retrograde amnesia, the forgetting of some recently acquired information. Lesions of the hippocampal circuit in man produce an amnestic syndrome. This clinicopathologic correlation was first appreciated by Milner and Falconer in a patient H.M., who underwent bilateral anterior temporal resections for intractable epilepsy. Postoperatively, H.M. had a dense and long-lasting amnestic syndrome. He has been studied over 30 years, and the amnesia persists undiminished. H.M. shows good capacity for formal reasoning and a normal I.Q., but a complete inability to master new facts, remember new acquaintances, or adjust to unfamiliar surroundings.

The clinical literature on amnesia suggests that bilateral lesions involving the hippocampus or medial dorsal thalamus are sufficient to produce the syndrome. (A transient or modality-specific deficit is often seen after unilateral lesions.) An example is the Korsakoff syndrome, a disorder seen most often in chronic alcoholics. It is due to involvement of limbic structures, particularly the mamillary nucleus and medial dorsal thalamus, from Wernicke's hemorrhagic encephalopathy. (Wernicke's disease is a thiamine deficiency disorder of the CNS.) The chronic syndrome is characterized by total anterograde amnesia, with a retrograde gradient of loss, and confabulation. A similar amnestic syndrome may occur from stroke, herpes simplex, encephalitis, or damage to the hippocampus from trauma or ischemia. The pyramidal cells of CA1 (Sommer's sector) are particularly vulnerable to hypoxic or ischemic injury. A recent case (R.B.) was described by Zola-Morgan, Squire, and co-workers, in which enduring amnesia resulted from a severe hypotensive episode. The pathology was largely restricted to CA1 pyramidal cells.

Cingulate Gyrus

The cingulate gyrus is a cortical structure which overlies the corpus callosum, continuous with the parahippocampal gyrus of the temporal lobe. Within it lies a longitudinal fiber bundle, the cingulum. The cingulate gyrus receives neocortical afferents, and limbic connections within the circuit of Papez. The anterior cingulate region is a limbic component of the frontal lobe, thought to be concerned with motivation. This region receives an afferent projection from the midbrain ventral tegmental area, a dopamine-bearing pathway (Fig. 8-22). The mesocortical dopamine system parallels the nigrostriatal tract, and is thought to have an influence on behavioral activation. One hypothesis suggests that some of the negative or *defect symptoms* of schizophrenia (flat affect, social withdrawal, lack of initiative) are related to the cingulate and dorsolateral prefrontal cortex, the target field of the mesocortical dopamine system. Surgical section of the anterior cingulate has an effect on behavior, particularly on the inhibitions of patients with chronic depression or severe anxiety disorders. This procedure (cingulotomy) is a kind of personality-altering surgery, or psychosurgery, a procedure which raises difficult ethical questions. As a treatment of last resort, it has helped some patients with disabling obsessive-compulsive behaviors, refractory to years of psychotherapy and medications.

The Amygdala

The amygdaloid nuclear complex is a gray matter mass in the anterior temporal lobe—a limbic structure derived from the basal ganglia. It

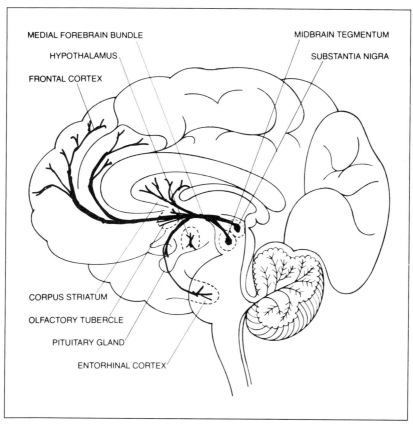

MEDIAL FOREBRAIN BUNDLE

HYPOTHALAMUS

FRONTAL CORTEX

MIDBRAIN TEGMENTUM

SUBSTANTIA NIGRA

CORPUS STRIATUM

OLFACTORY TUBERCLE

PITUITARY GLAND

ENTORHINAL CORTEX

FIGURE 8-22. Dopamine pathways of the forebrain. The neurons that contain dopamine have their cell bodies in two small regions of the midbrain: the substantia nigra and ventral tegmental area. The nigrostriatal pathway contains about 75 percent of the dopamine in the forebrain, and is part of the motor system. The other pathways have their origin in the ventral tegmental area, with projections to the nucleus accumbens (mesolimbic) and the frontal cortex (mesocortical). Dopamine is also found in the hypothalamus. (From L. Iversen, The chemistry of the brain. *Scientific American,* September 1979, p. 77, with permission.)

has two parts, a corticomedial and a basolateral nuclear group, and is thinly invested by the entorhinal cortex of the anterior temporal lobe. There are many sources of afferents to the amygdala, including the hypothalamus, septal area, brainstem, and cortex. Olfactory afferents terminate in the corticomedial nucleus, while cortical afferents favor the basolateral group. There are two efferent pathways. The stria terminalis follows the fornix and caudate, arching through the hemisphere to reach the septal area and hypothalamus. A ventral pathway goes directly across the uncus to the base of the brain, carrying information to the inferior frontal lobe, the diencephalon, and brainstem reticular core.

Stimulation of the amygdala in animals or in man evokes powerful emotional responses: anxiety, fear, and rage. The amygdala has a low threshold for the development of epilepsy. It can be "kindled." We can learn something from the ictal experiences of patients with temporal lobe epilepsy. A majority of such patients have a seizure focus in the limbic structures of the anterior temporal lobe (the amygdala and/ or hippocampus). Descriptions from such patients include the following: (1) An intense smell (olfactory aura) commonly precedes lapse of consciousness. It is usually unpleasant. (2) The aura may be emotional or visceral, an intense feeling which patients find hard to characterize. Consistent with the work on amygdala stimulation, anxiety and fear are most commonly reported. (3) A strange feeling of dissociation may be experienced, or a suggestion that the present moment is memorably familiar from the patient's past. This is known as déjà vu; perhaps it is expressed by the hippocampus. (4) Ictal aggression is probably quite rare; but grandiose delusions and ictal psychosis are occasionally seen. (5) A few patients have experienced pleasurable and frankly sexual sensations in association with their seizures.

Bilateral injury of the amygdala in animals produces a characteristic behavioral disorder: the Klüver-Bucy syndrome. Features include the triad of placidity, orality, and hypersexuality. Monkeys that have bilateral anterior temporal resection involving the amygdala lose their characteristic aggressive behavior, and become mild and tame. They put everything within their grasp into the mouth, as if they can no longer determine by looking whether an object is edible. They also become indiscriminate in their sexual behavior. They will approach and attempt to mount other animals of the same or opposite sex or of other species, and even inanimate objects. Aspects of the syndrome have been observed in human patients with destructive, bilateral anterior temporal lesions (e.g., herpes simplex encephalitis.)

Septal Area and Substantia Innominata

The septal area is difficult to define anatomically, due to its indistinct boundaries. It is that area anterior to the hypothalamus, underneath the frontal horn of the lateral ventricle, and adjacent to the septum pellucidum, from which the region derives its name. The precommissural fornix terminates here. The medial forebrain bundle, the principal monoamine pathway of the forebrain, traverses the septal area.

The medial septal nucleus is one of the places where Olds and Milner first reported the phenomenon of intracranial self-stimulation. In the rat, an implanted electrode in this location can be hooked up to a foot pedal, so that the animal can administer to himself a mild electric shock. Rats will push the bar continually, up to 5,000 times per hour, neglecting food and water, to pursue self-stimulation. Stimulation of this region in man results in a feeling of intense pleasure, reported as having a somewhat sexual quality. For this reason, the septal area and medial forebrain bundle are sometimes thought of as a "pleasure center" or reward system, a locus for positive reinforcement in behaviorist models of the nervous system.

The nucleus accumbens is the anterior part of the nuclear mass of the neostriatum (caudate and putamen). It lies along the lateral margin of the septal area. Like the caudate and putamen, it receives dopamine afferents from the midbrain, and contains a high concentration of dopamine receptors. Dopamine afferents come from the ventral tegmental area rather than from the substantia nigra. Its input-output relations define the nucleus accumbens as a part of the limbic system, rather than the motor system. This is one of the places where antipsychotic drugs may have an effect on delusions and hallucinations in schizophrenia.

The nucleus of Meynert lies in an adjacent region of the basal forebrain, the substantia innominata. The substantia innominata is the unnamed substance under the anterior commissure. The medial septal nucleus and basal nucleus of Meynert contain a majority of large cholinergic neurons. These nuclei form a cholinergic projection system (Fig. 8-23): The septal nucleus gives rise to a cholinergic pathway to the hippocampus (septohippocampal pathway). The basal nucleus provides an extensive cholinergic projection to the neocortex. Substantial cell loss in this region has been described in Alzheimer's disease. Attempts to treat the memory and attention deficits in Alzheimer's disease have utilized drugs which enhance cholinergic synaptic function.

Integrated Function of the Limbic System

In 1928, Phillip Bard did a study of the effects of CNS lesions on behavior in the cat. A transection of the nervous system which preserved the caudal hypothalamus and brainstem produced a phenomenon known as *sham rage*. In response to handling, the cat would produce a dramatic emotional display. The cat would bare his claws and teeth, arch his back, spit, and hiss: the picture of a terrific fury.

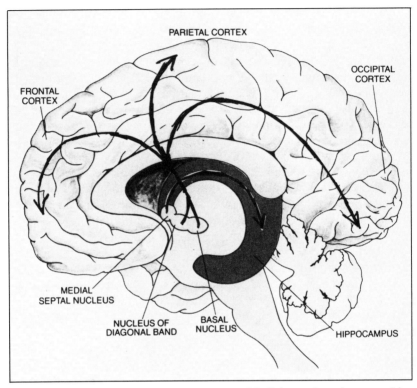

FIGURE 8-23. Cholinergic projection system. Medial septal nucleus provides the cholinergic innervation of the hippocampus. Basal nucleus of Meynert is the source of neocortical projections. A more detailed map is found in Figure 3-7. (From R.J. Wurtman, Alzheimer's disease. *Scientific American* January 1985, p. 73, with permission.)

The response was superficial and disconnected; there was no directed attack. When the stimulation was over, the response would quickly subside. The hypothalamus and reticular formation can command a range of primitive responses, including coughing, vomiting, yawning, crying, sexual arousal, and control of the pituitary and autonomic nervous system. The limbic system is necessary, however, to provide oversight and give these responses a context and behavioral relevance.

Limbic structures project inward to the hypothalamus and brainstem reticular core. The septal area directly adjoins the hypothalamus along the medial forebrain bundle. The hippocampus projects to the hypothalamus and septal area through the fornix. Centrally directed connections of the amygdala include the stria terminalis, and the ventral pathway across the uncus to the thalamus and brainstem.

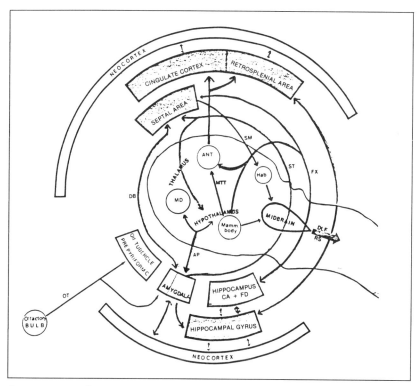

FIGURE 8-24. The interconnections of the limbic system: The hypothalamus and brainstem control the viscera and internal milieu. Neocortical systems process and analyze information regarding our relation to the external world. The limbic system (*stippled*) can be considered a network of structures that manages the interface between these environments.

The hippocampus includes Ammon's horn (CA) and the fascia dentata (FD). The hippocampal gyrus includes the entorhinal area. FX designates the fornix; ST, the stria terminalis; and SM, the stria medullaris. The dorsal longitudinal fasciculus (DLF) and reticulospinal tract (RS) are descending brainstem pathways. Hab = habenula; MD and ANT = thalamic nuclei, AP = ansa peduncularis; OT = olfactory tract; DB = diagonal band; MTT = mammillothalamic tract.

The figure is from a 1982 lecture by Dr. Marsel Mesulam, and does not include the extensive connections of the basal nucleus reviewed above.

Limbic structures also enjoy extensive bidirectional connections with the cerebral cortex. The basolateral nuclear group of the amygdala projects to the neocortex of the orbital frontal lobe, temporal lobe, and insula. The entorhinal cortex of the temporal lobe enjoys regional corticocortical connections. The cingulate gyrus has bidirectional connections throughout its length with the neocortex of the cerebral convexity. Cholinergic projections from the basal forebrain influence cortical processing.

An overview of the limbic system begins to emerge (Fig. 8-24). Limbic structures ring the medial wall of the cerebral hemispheres, interconnected by the circuit of Papez. They are interposed between the hypothalamus, the "visceral brain" which regards the internal milieu, and the neocortex, which handles information on the external environment. This location is strategic. Limbic structures process and monitor emotional aspects of experience and direct emotional responses. Together with the frontal lobe, they help us understand the behavioral consequences of our internal needs. They also select and mark external events meaningful to us for memory.

It is therefore not surprising that diseases affecting the limbic system have visceral and behavioral manifestations. Tumors or epilepsy in limbic system structures can have neuroendocrine or autonomic effects, and commonly produce an alteration in personality. Lesions in the limbic system pathways discussed above produce disturbances of emotion, motivation, or memory.

BIBLIOGRAPHY

Cortical Functions

Geschwind, N. Disconnection syndromes in animals and man. *Brain* 88 : 237–294, 585–644, 1965.
Geschwind, N. Specializations of the human brain. *Sci. Am.* 241 : 180–201, 1979.
Mountcastle, V.B. An Organizing Principal for Cerebral Function. In F.O. Schmitt and F.G. Worden (eds.), *The Neurosciences: Fourth Study Program.* Cambridge, Mass.: MIT Press, 1979. Pp. 21–42.
Penfield, W., and Jasper, H. *Epilepsy and the Functional Anatomy of the Human Brain.* Boston: Little, Brown, 1954.

Limbic System and Behavior

Klüver, H., and Bucy, P. Preliminary analysis of functions of the temporal lobe in monkeys, *Arch. Neurol. Psychiatry* 42 : 979, 1939.
Mesulam, M. *Principles of Behavioral Neurology.* Philadelphia: Davis, 1985.
Mesulam, M. Neural Substrates of Behavior. In A.M. Nicholi (ed.), *The New Harvard Guide to Psychiatry.* Cambridge, Mass.: Belknap Press, 1988. Pp. 91–128.
Squire, L. Mechanisms of memory. *Science* 232 : 1612–1619, 1986.

PART IV

Vulnerabilities of the Nervous System

CHAPTER 9

Cerebrospinal Fluid, Intracranial Dynamics, and Central Nervous System Tumors

This chapter considers the physics of the intracranial compartment and the composition of its principal humor: the cerebrospinal fluid (CSF). Cerebrospinal fluid buffers the brain against trauma. The exclusion of solutes by the blood-brain barrier is an important defense mechanism against toxins or metabolic change. Cellular and chemical responses of the CSF are helpful clues in the diagnosis of central nervous system (CNS) disorders. Brain edema, hydrocephalus, or an expanding mass can elevate the intracranial pressure, and may compromise nervous system function. These subjects form the basis for a discussion of the physiology of brain and spinal tumors.

THE CEREBROSPINAL FLUID CIRCULATION

The brain is roughly 80 percent water. The proportion of water is higher in nervous tissues than in other parts of the body. This includes cell water in neurons and supporting cells, and brain extra-cellular fluid. Another 75 cc of fluid lies in the intracranial blood vessels. In addition, the nervous system maintains a sizeable reservoir of CSF. The ventricular system contains 50 cc of CSF, while another 25 to 50 cc invest the nervous system in the craniospinal subarachnoid space, and the cisterns of the intracranial compartment (Fig. 9-1).

Cerebrospinal fluid is secreted in the choroid plexus, most of it in the paired lateral ventricles (Fig. 9-2). The C-shaped lateral ventricles are each connected to the third ventricle via the intraventricular foramen of Monro. The single third ventricle lies in the midline, between the paired nuclei of the thalamus. The aqueduct of Sylvius connects the third ventricle with the fourth, which lies in the posterior fossa between the cerebellum and brainstem. Paired lateral foramina

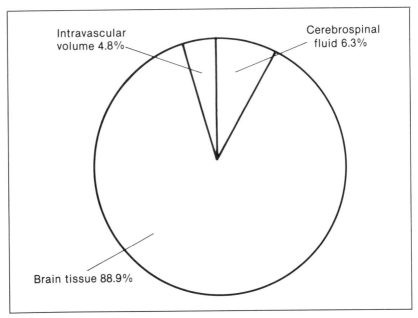

FIGURE 9-1. Contents of the intracranial compartment.

of Luschka, and the single midline foramen of Magendie open into the basal cistern, or cisterna magna. The choroid plexus protrudes into the ventricles, and contains a network of fine vessels. Its stroma secretes CSF at a fixed rate, largely independent of back pressure in the system. The secretion of CSF involves a carbonic anhydrase dependent–mechanism. The stroma of the choroid plexus can calcify with age, a change often observed on skull films or computed tomography (CT). When CSF leaves the ventricles via the foramina of Luschka and Magendie, it joins the subarachnoid space which surrounds the CNS.

Cerebrospinal fluid in the subarachnoid space invests penetrating arteries as they enter the brain parenchyma. This extension of the subarachnoid space around small arteries is known as the Virchow-Robin space. Figure 9-3, A, illustrates the normal relations of the Virchow-Robin space. The CSF also permeates the subarachnoid space surrounding the spinal cord, its ligaments, and segmental nerve roots. Cerebrospinal fluid pools in the caudal sac beneath the termination of the spinal cord at L1, where it bathes the trailing lumbosacral roots of the cauda equina.

Cerebrospinal fluid is resorbed into the dural sinuses. Specializations of arachnoid, the arachnoid granulations, develop within the principal venous sinuses. Figure 9-4 shows how arachnoid granula-

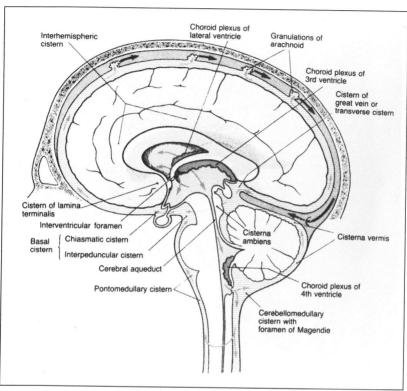

FIGURE 9-2. The circulation of CSF. Cerebrospinal fluid is produced in the ventricles, in the choroid plexus. Through the foramina of the fourth ventricle, CSF enters the cisterns and subarachnoid space. (Reprinted by permission from Duus, P.: *Topical Diagnosis in Neurology*, Thieme Medical Publishers, New York, 1983.)

tions, each resembling a bunch of grapes, line the inferomedial margin of the superior sagittal sinus. The arachnoid granulations allow CSF to leave the subarachnoid spaces and flow into the venous system through a "one-way valve." The pressure-dependent extrusion of CSF is a bulk flow mechanism. There is no separation or filtration of CSF; everything leaves together whenever ambient pressure in the subarachnoid space exceeds the venous pressure in the venous sinus.

The rate of production of CSF is 0.35 ml/min, or roughly 540 ml/day. This is 4 to 5 times the capacity of the system, so that the CSF in the ventricles and subarachnoid spaces is turned over 4 to 5 times per day. Under steady-state conditions, CSF resorption is also 0.35 ml/min into the venous sinuses. Figure 9-5 illustrates the equilibrium between the

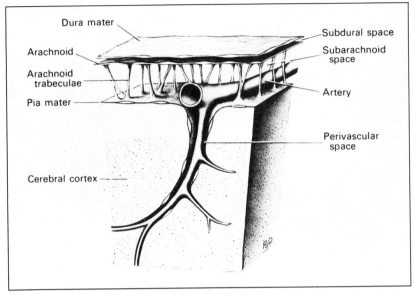

A

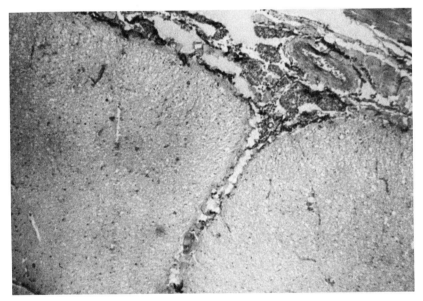

B

FIGURE 9-3. A. Drawing illustrates the perivascular or Virchow-Robin space, an extension of the subarachnoid space. (From M.B. Carpenter, *Core Text of Neuroanatomy* [3rd ed.]. Baltimore: Williams & Wilkins, 1986, p. 12, with permission.) B. Stained section taken from a patient with carcinomatous meningitis demonstrates malignant cells in the subarachnoid space, extending into the perivascular space.

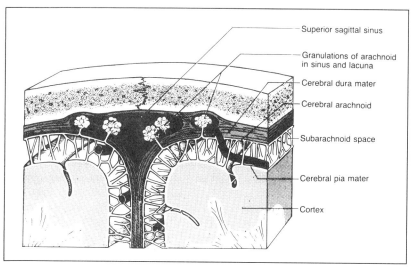

Superior sagittal sinus

Granulations of arachnoid
in sinus and lacuna

Cerebral dura mater

Cerebral arachnoid

Subarachnoid space

Cerebral pia mater

Cortex

FIGURE 9-4. Coronal section through the superior sagittal sinus. Arachnoid granulations extend into the sinus, and are a port of exit for CSF. (Reprinted by permission from Duus, P.: *Topical Diagnosis in Neurology*, Thieme Medical Publishers, New York, 1983.)

rate of CSF formation and resorption, a principal determinant of the intracranial pressure.

The Cerebrospinal Fluid

The primary function of CSF is to support and protect the brain. The buoyancy of the brain reduces gravitational forces on the tissue, and the fluid reservoir acts as a mechanical buffer. The brain is soft in consistency and would otherwise be easily bruised against the petrous bone, sphenoid wing, and olfactory groove.

The CSF resembles an ultrafiltrate of plasma. Its protein content is lower, less than 50 mg/100 ml total protein. Cerebrospinal fluid proteins include native immunoglobulins produced by plasma cells inside the intracranial compartment. Some polypeptide hormones and biogenic amine metabolites can also be in solution. Cerebrospinal fluid is very slightly acidic relative to blood, as some carbon dioxide is liberated by the brain from the metabolism of glucose. Glucose and amino acids are actively transported into the brain. CSF glucose is roughly two-thirds of the serum glucose averaged over the preceding hours.

In health the CSF is relatively acellular; it is strikingly abnormal to have as many as five white cells in a cubic millimeter of CSF. Spun samples contain a few mononuclear cells, and occasional arachnoid

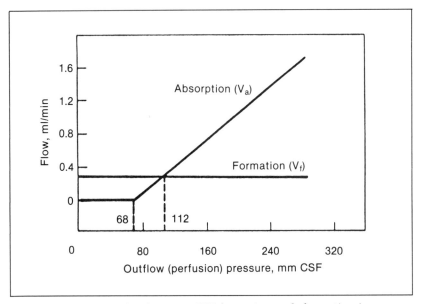

FIGURE 9-5. Relationship between CSF formation and absorption in man determines the intracranial pressure at equilibrium. The rate of CSF formation is nearly constant; the rate of absorption increases with pressure once the "one-way valve" of the arachnoid villus opens, here shown at a pressure of 68 mm CSF. (From R.W.P. Cutler, L. Page, J. Galicich, and G.V. Watters, Formation and absorption of cerebral spinal fluid in man. *Brain* 91 : 707–720, 1968, with permission.)

cells. Analysis of CSF is useful in diagnosis, and essential to the prompt diagnosis of bacterial meningitis. Cerebrospinal fluid can be obtained by needle puncture at a lumbar interspace, caudal to the termination of the spinal cord at L1. Normal CSF findings are listed in Table 9-1. A look at the spun fluid is useful to distinguish subarachnoid hemorrhage from a traumatic tap. A supernatant yellow with protein or heme-deprived pigment (xanthochromia) suggests recent hemorrhage.

Protein may be elevated in cases of intracranial tumor or infection. Patients with disease involving proximal parts of the peripheral nervous system may weep protein into the subarachnoid space. A CSF protein in excess of 500 mg/100 ml suggests an obstruction to the spinal subarachnoid circulation with stasis in the caudal sac. Patients with inflammatory or demyelinating diseases may have abnormal immunoglobulins in the spinal fluid. A gamma globulin in excess of 13 percent of total protein, or an oligoclonal banding pattern on immunoelectrophoresis suggests inflammatory or demyelinating disease. Glucose may be reduced in active meningitis, due to abnormal

TABLE 9-1. Cerebrospinal Fluid Findings in Selected Neurologic Disorders

Disorder	Gross Appearance	Pressure (mm H_2O)	Cells (cu mm)	Protein (mg/100 ml)
Normal values	Clear	70–150	None	20–50
Bacterial meningitis	Cloudy	› 200	› 1000 (poly-morphonu-clear WBCs)	Elevated
Tuberculous meningitis	Cloudy	› 200	10–500 (lympho-cytes)	Elevated
Viral meningitis	Clear	Normal	0–200	20–100
Herpes simplex encephalitis	Clear	Normal to slightly elevated	10–200 lymphocytes, RBCs	50–150
Subarachnoid hemorrhage	Bloody, xantho-chromic	Elevated	300–20,000 RBCs	50 + 4/1,000 RBCs
Parameningeal focus of infection	Clear	Normal	0–50 lymphocytes	20–100
Brain tumor	Clear	Normal or elevated	0–4	Elevated
Carcinomatous meningitis	Clear or thick	Slightly elevated	4–50, tumor cells	100–200

transport into the CSF. A glucose under 40 mg/100 ml suggests acute bacterial meningitis or active chronic infection.

Intracranial infection is reflected in the CSF formula, particularly the nature and vigor of the cellular response. In acute bacterial meningitis (in an immunologically normal host) a vigorous polymorphonuclear response is seen. Cell counts usually exceed 1,000 leukocytes. Chronic meningitis or opportunistic infection may have a smaller, predominantly mononuclear response. In viral infections, CSF cell counts under 500 are the rule, and polymorphonuclear leukocytes are unusual after the first 1 to 2 days. Cytologic examination may disclose tumor cells in patients with leptomeningeal cancer.

THE BLOOD-BRAIN BARRIER

The blood-brain barrier was discovered in the nineteenth century by Paul Ehrlich. When he injected trypan blue into the circulation, he noticed that the brain did not take up the stain found in most other

organs. Cerebral arteries differ from systemic arteries in their imper-
meability to large molecules, a difference often conceptualized as
a barrier. The blood-brain barrier is not, in fact, an actual physical
barrier, but rather an elaborate system for brain extracellular fluid
(ECF) homeostasis. This system includes (1) specializations in brain-
penetrating arterioles and capillaries; (2) the choroid plexus and
arachnoid granulations, which form the interface between the systemic circulation and CSF; and (3) the pial and ependymal lining
which separates the brain ECF from fluid in the ventricles and subarachnoid space. The blood-brain barrier is the key to understanding
the distribution kinetics of drugs and other small molecules which
may enter the brain.

A closer look at its component parts demonstrates the importance
of specialized anatomy at the blood-brain, blood-CSF, and brain-CSF
interfaces. (1) Brain capillaries, in contrast to systemic capillaries, are
characterized by endothelial tight junctions, which impede diffusion
out of the lumen. In addition, glial foot processes wrap end arterioles
and capillaries to ensure a tight seal (Fig. 9-6). Glucose and amino
acids required for CNS metabolism are transported across this membrane by a carrier-mediated transport mechanism. (2) The choroid
plexus and the arachnoid granulations form an interface between the
circulation and the CSF reservoir, controlling secretion and absorption
of CSF. (3) The internal and external surfaces of the brain are lined
with specialized tissue where they contact the CSF. The ependyma
affords a layer of protection to the periventricular neuropil. The pial-
glial membrane forms the internal limiting membrane of the subarachnoid space.

Molecular size and polarity are the principal determinants of solute
access to brain tissue. Sucrose, molecular weight 360, crosses easily
from the circulation; inulin (mol wt 5,000) does not. Plasma proteins
do not enter the brain to any appreciable extent. The concentration of
albumin in the CSF is less than 0.5 percent of that in serum. Bilirubin
is likewise excluded from the adult brain. Consequently, the brain is
not normally icteric, even in deeply jaundiced individuals. In the
premature infant, for whom the barrier has not yet matured, high
serum concentrations of bilirubin can penetrate and injure the brain,
resulting in a condition known as kernicterus. Polar molecules are
excluded by the blood-brain barrier. Consequently CO_2 diffuses, but
HCO_3 does not pass. Dihydroxyphenylalanine (L-dopa) crosses,
whereas dopamine, a polar molecule, does not. Highly lipid-soluble
molecules such as halothane, ethanol, pentobarbital, chlorampheni-
col, and vitamin A diffuse easily into the brain.

The circumventricular organs are a collection of specialized structures adjacent to the ventricles and subarachnoid space. The pineal,

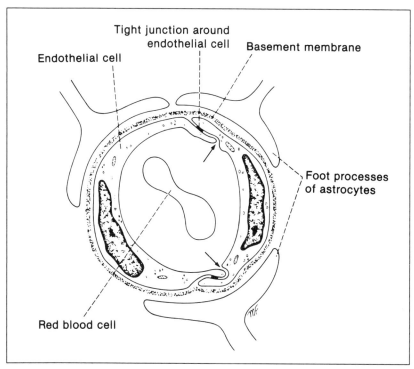

FIGURE 9-6. Structural components of the blood-brain barrier: The brain capillary is ensheathed by astrocyte foot processes, and tight junctions are present at the apposition of endothelial cells. The basement membrane holds the endothelium together, and helps maintain its tubular form. (From R. Snell, *Clinical Neuroanatomy for Medical Students* [2nd ed.]. Boston: Little, Brown, 1987, p. 336, with permission.)

subforniceal organ, subcommisural organ, median eminence, and area postrema are shown in Figure 9-7. In each of these regions the blood-brain barrier is permeable to a wider range of substances. The area postrema has chemoreceptors which monitor the blood gases, serum bicarbonate, and solutes normally excluded from the brain. The median eminence and organ vasculosum of the lamina terminalis are involved in peptide secretion and neuroendocrine function.

The blood-brain barrier may be altered in disease. In meningitis or in brain adjacent to a tumor or abscess, there is increased diffusion of large molecules, including antibiotics and antineoplastic agents. This diffusion, however, is not reliable enough to be an access for treatment. It is preferable to treat CNS diseases with drugs that penetrate well. Imaging techniques capitalize on regional changes in the blood-brain barrier that occur in disease. Intravenous (IV) contrast used

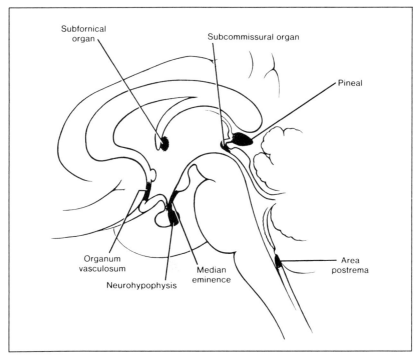

FIGURE 9-7. The circumventricular organs: specialized areas where gaps in the blood-brain barrier allow the nervous system to sample nondiffusible substances in the circulation. (From M.B. Carpenter and J. Sutin, *Human Neuroanatomy* [8th ed.]. Baltimore: Williams & Wilkins, 1985, p. 23, with permission.)

during computed tomography (CT) scan will leak out around a cerebral infarction or CNS neoplasm. Recently there has been interest in forcing a transient opening in the blood-brain barrier at the capillary level with osmotic plasma expanders. This experimental technique may enable large molecules to permeate the barrier for therapeutic purposes.

BRAIN EDEMA

Many common diseases (tumor, stroke, cerebral trauma) foster the accumulation of excess water in CNS tissues. Brain edema is hazardous because it causes brain tissue to expand, acting like a space-occupying lesion. Brain edema has been classified into three types according to mechanism: vasogenic edema, cytotoxic edema, and interstitial edema. Vasogenic edema is highly sensitive to therapy, and treatment of edema in cases of tumor can result in dramatic clinical change. Edema impairs the function of nervous tissue, and may even contribute to cellular injury.

Vasogenic edema is due to abnormal permeability of the blood-brain barrier (Fig. 9-8). The tight junctions of endothelial cells in brain capillaries leak, allowing a transudate, or plasma filtrate, to enter the extracellular compartment. It is not clear how excess fluid and plasma proteins impair nervous function. There is probably some tamponade of myelinated axons, and perhaps a change in the ionic properties of the membrane as well. Vasogenic edema is common around brain tumors. Edema may involve peritumoral white matter to an extreme degree. Osmotic agents such as mannitol help draw water back into the intravascular space. With prolonged use they may diffuse into the brain and lose their effectiveness. Corticosteroids improve the apposition at endothelial tight junctions and are highly effective at counteracting edema formation.

Cytoxic edema is a response to cell injury and tissue necrosis. As in any injury of soft tissue, injured cells swell and take up water. The cells are unable to pump sodium and water out. Such swelling is a minor problem with a contusion or bruise in a limb, but presents a major problem in the intracranial compartment. Cytotoxic edema is present after ischemic necrosis and may be present after trauma. This kind of edema does not respond well to osmotic agents or steroids. Pure interstitial edema occurs infrequently, most commonly with hydrocephalus. Brain edema observed on the CT scan in the absence of hydrocephalus is usually a combination of vasogenic and cytotoxic edema in varying degrees.

INTRACRANIAL DYNAMICS

The pressure in the intracranial compartment can be measured during lumbar puncture in the standard lateral decubitus position. A manometer is connected to the needle within the spinal subarachnoid space, and the system is allowed to reach open equilibrium. The normal range of CSF pressure is 65 to 150 mm H_2O. Intracranial pressure (ICP) is position-dependent, reflecting the height of the sagittal sinus over the venous angle (right atrium). This fact reflects the need for a slight pressure gradient maintaining CSF egress into the venous sinuses. Intracranial pressure will rise as new fluid is produced until it just exceeds intracranial venous pressure (jugular venous pressure). Cerebrospinal pressure will drain as jugular pressure falls. Intracranial pressure is thus lowest in the upright posture, increased in the supine position, and elevated still further with the head dependent. Cough,

234

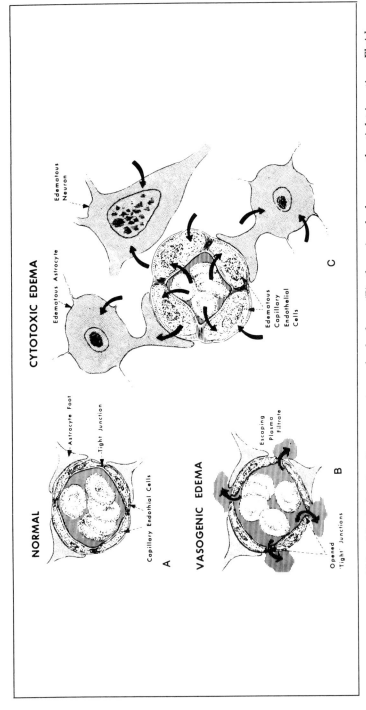

FIGURE 9-8. A. Normal blood-brain barrier. In vasogenic cerebral edema (B), there is a leak across the tight junction. Fluid escapes into the extracellular space. With cytotoxic edema (C), there is diffuse swelling of endothelia, glia, and neuronal cells, and the extracellular space contracts (From R. Fishman, Brain edema. *N. Engl. J. Med.* 293 : 707, 1975. Reprinted by permission of the *New England Journal of Medicine.*)

abdominal pressure, exhalation, and the Valsalva maneuver transiently increase intracranial pressure. (This phenomenon can be observed during lumbar puncture.)

The cranial vault is a rigid container, with a capacity of 1,500 to 1,600 cc. The brain occupies 1,400 cc, which allows for 100 to 125 cc of CSF, 70 to 80 cc of blood in the intravascular compartment, plus a few thoughts and vapors. The brain is a soft, but relatively noncompressible solid. The capacity of the system to accommodate an additional volume load is thus very limited. An expanding mass to 50 to 70 cc can be tolerated by displacing fluid from the ventricles (see Fig. 9-1). Past this point, any further expansion must displace brain tissue. Thus, the intracranial compartment has a limited capacity to accommodate a volume load and a rapid increase in pressure when overstuffed. Figure 9-9 illustrates the pressure volume curve in man measured from monitoring spontaneous variations in the neurosurgical intensive care unit (ICU). Beyond a particular "breakpoint" for the system, which varies from individual to individual, the pressure increase is exponential.

Constant monitoring of the ICP in the neurologic-neurosurgical ICU demonstrates that pressure is rarely constant over time. Transient elevations in pressure accompany peaks in arterial pressure (in systole). Pressure is also increased somewhat during expiration. Significant transient elevations lasting minutes are observed in patients with raised ICP. These transient pressure waves (Lundberg waves or plateau waves) are shown in recordings from ICP monitoring (Fig. 9-10). The patient's clinical status may change dramatically during such transient elevations in pressure.

What problem is posed by a rise in ICP above 150 mm H_2O? If the load is evenly distributed, the brain tolerates pressures of 300 to 500 mm H_2O. Modest increases (up to 200%) are apparently not detrimental to the nervous system. A greater problem occurs at the interface in the intracranial compartment, where brain and other tissues meet. One such place is the eye. The optic nerve is an extension of the CNS invested in a dural sheath, and intracranial pressure is transmitted along it. Intraocular pressure is determined by local mechanisms. Papilledema occurs when a sustained increase in ICP is transmitted to the optic nerve head. Within 18 to 24 hours, this becomes evident as disc swelling and edema. With chronically elevated pressures (weeks to months), some loss of vision results from chronic edema of the optic disc and nerve fiber layer.

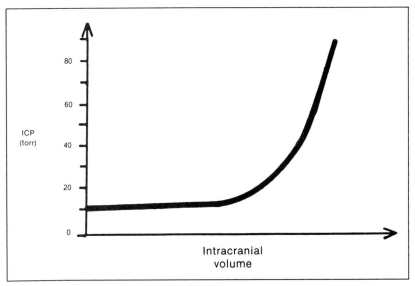

FIGURE 9-9. Response of intracranial pressure (ICP) to a volume load. As a volume of fluid is added to the intracranial compartment, pressure rises steeply once the compensatory limits of the system are exceeded. (From H.M. Shapiro, Intracranial hypertension. *Anesthesiology* 43 : 447, 1975, with permission.)

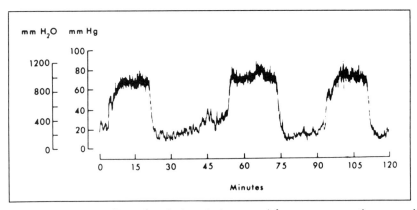

FIGURE 9-10. Recording of variations in intracranial pressure over time, monitored from a patient with a brain tumor. Three plateau waves (Lundberg A waves) are evident. (From N. Lundberg, Continuous recording and control of ventricular fluid pressure in neurosurgical practice. *Acta Psychiatr. Neurol. Scand.* [*Suppl.*] 36 : 1, 1960.)

Exceedingly high ICPs begin to threaten cerebral perfusion. Cerebral perfusion pressure has two determinants, systemic arterial pressure and ICP. Cerebral perfusion pressure is simply the excess of arterial pressure over ICP. Mean arterial pressure is generally 80 to 100 mm Hg (1,000–1,300 mm H_2O). As intracranial pressure increases, arterial pressure rises somewhat to compensate (Cushing's reflex). With an increase in ICP above 1,000 mm H_2O, the cerebral circulation may collapse. A pressure increase of this degree is inconsistent with survival.

Compartment Syndrome: Brain Herniation

If it is uniformly distributed, raised ICP will be tolerated within a limited range, as described above. A more serious problem results from an imbalanced expansion of brain in one part of the intracranial compartment. The tentorium and falx divide the intracranial space into subcompartments, as illustrated in Figure 9-11. These fibrous structures are firm and tethered, and thus movement is restricted. An imbalanced, or regional expansion, can force the extrusion, or herniation, of brain from one subcompartment to another. Herniation of the cingulate gyrus under the falx to accommodate an expanding mass on one side will cause damage to the cingulate gyrus, a relatively subtle clinical syndrome. A greater problem occurs with medial displacement of the temporal lobe into the tentorium.

The tentorium is attached to the falx at the straight sinus, and is tethered anteriorly at the clinoid process (the pituitary fossa). The relations of the tentorium are important: the width accommodates the midbrain and is somewhat variable among individuals. Extrusion of the uncus of the temporal lobe into the tentorial incisura (uncal herniation) may compress the midbrain, causing brainstem injury and a fatal outcome. The third nerve is trapped against the posterior cerebral artery as the temporal lobe advances, so that its compromise is an early clinical sign. Transtentorial herniation and brainstem compression are a frequent cause of death in patients with an expanding intracranial mass.

If an expanding mass develops within the posterior fossa, the cerebellar tonsils can extrude through the foramen magnum. Cerebellar tonsillar herniation causes a fatal syndrome if the lower medulla is compressed. Pressure alone is infrequently the cause of mortality in patients with an intracranial mass. Rather it is displacement of brain and compromise of vital structures in the reticular core that is the proximate cause of death.

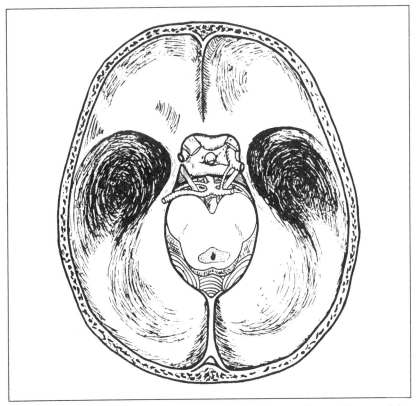

FIGURE 9-11. The tentorial opening is illustrated in this figure. The cranial cap and forebrain have been removed and you are looking into the floor of the anterior and middle cranial fossae. This perspective is seen when the brain is removed post mortem. Note the relationship between the exiting third nerve, the posterior cerebral artery, and the petroclinoid ligament. (From F. Plum and J. Posner, *Stupor and Coma* [3rd ed.]. Philadelphia: Davis, 1985, p. 90, with permission.)

Hydrocephalus

Hydrocephalus ("water on the brain") is caused by an excess volume of CSF, resulting in distention of the ventricular system. Three mechanisms are described. In a freely communicating system, there may be oversecretion of CSF, resulting in excess accumulation. Alternatively, there may be impaired absorption, a phenomenon which is far more common. Either variety is a type of *communicating hydrocephalus*; the system is open to the free passage of CSF. An obstruction to CSF flow can cause noncommunicating, or *obstructive hydrocephalus* (Table 9-2).

Oversecretion of CSF is rare. The system can normally accommodate a two- to threefold increase in CSF production before compensatory

TABLE 9-2. Hydrocephalus

Type	Mechanism/Variety
Communicating	Overproduction of CSF (rare)
	Choroid plexus tumor
	Impaired absorption
	Posttraumatic hydrocephalus
	Normal-pressure hydrocephalus
Noncommunicating	Obstruction to flow
	Aqueductal stenosis
	Posterior fossa malformation
	Tumor

mechanisms are overwhelmed. Only in choroid plexus tumors of infancy is there such an abundant hypersecretion of CSF. Impaired absorption is the more common mechanism for communicating hydrocephalus. The arachnoid granulations can become congested with fibrin or protein after meningitis or subarachnoid hemorrhage. Idiopathic communicating hydrocephalus occurs sometimes among older patients, associated with ventricular pressures in the normal range. The syndrome of normal-pressure hydrocephalus is of considerable interest as a reversible cause of dementia and/or gait disorder in the elderly.

Subtotal or partial obstruction of the CSF system at the aqueduct, the fourth ventricular outflow, or at the foramen of Monro will result in a pressure gradient across the obstruction, and increased pressure is transmitted throughout the system. Production of CSF will continue against a pressure gradient. Total obstruction causes acute hydrocephalus: a rapid distention of the system over hours, raised pressure, displacement of brain, and a clinical deterioration.

Benign Intracranial Hypertension

Symptoms and signs of intracranial hypertension sometimes occur in the absence of a space-occupying lesion. Some degree of brain edema may be present; the CT scan often demonstrates increased brain water and compression of the ventricular system. Pressures are commonly in the range of 200 to 500 mm H_2O. Headache may bring the patient to the physician, though the condition can be entirely asymptomatic! (Recall that modest pressure elevation does not embarrass brain function.) Visual loss may occur with time from the chronically elevated pressure and papilledema. This condition is known as *benign intracranial hypertension* (pseudotumor cerebri). Its cause is not well understood. Obesity appears to be a risk factor, and female patients outnumber

TABLE 9-3. Treatment of Raised Intracranial Pressure

Treatment	Reduces	Strategy
Corticosteroids	ECF	Reduce vasogenic brain edema
Urea, mannitol	ECF, ICF	Dehydrate brain, reduce edema
Diuretics	ECF, CSF	Reduce edema, CSF production
Hyperventilation	Blood volume	Induce vasoconstriction
Barbiturates	Blood volume	Reduce pressure waves
CSF diversion	CSF	Treat hydrocephalus
Craniotomy		Open skull, remove tissue

Key: ECF = extracellular fluid; ICF = intracellular fluid; CSF = cerebrospinal fluid.

males. In some cases, it can be related to medications (tetracyclines or hypervitaminosis A) or endocrine disturbance. Lumbar puncture with removal of 15 to 20 cc of CSF is sometimes curative, allowing the pressure to "reset" in the normal range. In patients who do not correct with lumbar puncture, medical management of intracranial hypertension is indicated to conserve vision.

Treatment of Raised Intracranial Pressure

It is sometimes necessary to treat raised intracranial pressure for the reasons outlined above. The avenues of approach to the management of elevated ICP are outlined in Table 9-3. Even in combination, the existing treatments are often inadequate. Corticosteroids and osmotic agents, such as urea and mannitol, are administered in order to decrease tissue water and reduce brain edema. Edema is a significant contributor to raised ICP. Diuretics, such as furosemide and acetazolamide, are occasionally useful. Acetazolamide, a carbonic anhydrase inhibitor, specifically reduces the secretion of CSF, and decreases the volume of fluid in the CSF compartment. Decreasing the carbon dioxide partial pressure (P_{CO_2}) by forced hyperventilation will reduce the volume of blood in the intravascular space, and temporarily lower the ICP. This is a useful approach for rapid lowering of pressure in an emergency, but may be counterproductive if continued for days. Barbiturates have an effect on autoregulation. In addition, they reduce tissue metabolic demand, and blunt spontaneous pressure waves. If these maneuvers fail to reduce the pressure and volume in the intracranial compartment, surgical treatment may be necessary. Diversion of CSF through a ventricular catheter can be particularly helpful if there is hydrocephalus. Sometimes craniotomy and decompression are necessary as a treatment of last resort.

PRIMARY BRAIN TUMOR

Tumors originate in nervous tissues with surprising frequency. An estimated 10,000 new cases are seen annually in hospitals in the United States. The presenting clinical features are a function of size and anatomic location. The natural history and clinical behavior, however, reflect the cell type of origin. A helpful perspective on the problem of brain tumor thus derives from an understanding of the biologic "roots" of the common intracranial neoplasms.

The cellular composition of the brain includes neuronal elements and supporting cells. Neuronal tumors are infrequent in medical practice. Glial elements give rise to a family of tumors: the astrocytoma, oligodendroglioma, and the malignant glioma. These are common, infiltrating, and notoriously heterogeneous. Their classification by histologic grade of malignancy may seem arbitrary. Nonetheless, the distinction between the low-grade astrocytoma and the grade III or IV glioblastoma is useful, when their clinical behavior is considered. The Schwann cells of the peripheral nervous system can become neoplastic also. These are the principal cell type of the acoustic neuroma, and participate in the growth of neurofibromas. Peripheral nervous system tumors tend to be more tractable.

The meninges are composed of connective tissue, and specialized ependymal cells border the ventricles. The meningiomas are connective tissue tumors, distantly related to other soft tissue sarcomas. They tend to be benign and encapsulated, although a wide range of behavior is observed. Ependymal tumors are most often seen in adults in the caudal spinal canal (the filum terminale). Lymphomas may originate within the nervous system, particularly in immunocompromised patients. Midline structures present in embryogenesis give rise to various teratomas, chordomas, and the Rathke's pouch tumor (craniopharyngioma). Small foci of pituitary adenoma are surprisingly common at general autopsy.

Cushing's experience (Table 9-4) gives a rough idea about the incidence of various tumors in a neurosurgical referral practice. It greatly understates the number of CNS metastases seen today in a busy general hospital.

Presentation

Tumors of the intracranial compartment produce general symptoms and signs related to altered intracranial dynamics, and specific focal signs related to their location. They usually present as a subacute or chronic disorder, evolving over weeks to months. Of the general symptoms, headache is the most frequent (75%), and is related to

TABLE 9-4. Incidence of Various Types of Intracranial Tumors

Tumor	Number	Percent
Gliomas	862	43.0
Meningiomas	271	14.0
Pituitary adenomas	360	18.0
Acoustic neuromas	176	9.0
Metastatic	85	4.0
Congenital	113	5.5
Blood vessel tumors	41	2.0
Miscellaneous	115	
Total	2,023	100

Source: H. Cushing, *Intracranial Tumors*. Springfield, Ill.: Thomas, 1932.

traction on the meninges and vessels. As you might predict, headache varies with posture. It may be less prominent with activity and worse during supine bed rest, such as to wake the patient from sleep. Pain is increased by bending, coughing, straining, or Valsalva maneuver, efforts that transiently raise intracranial pressure. Nausea and vomiting (present in 20–30% of patients) may be due to traction on structures in the floor of the fourth ventricle. Papilledema is not always seen with CNS tumors, although pressures above 150 mm H_2O can be recorded in 75 percent of patients. Seizures occur in 35 percent of supratentorial tumors and may be focal. They occur most often with vascular tumors near the cortical band, and somewhat less often with the rapidly infiltrating glial tumors. Mental status changes are often present, a manifestation of region cerebral dysfunction.

Specific features of location give the tumor syndrome its focal signature. Patients with frontal lobe tumors, for instance, are characteristically fatuous, irritable, uninhibited, and apathetic, and may have gait trouble and urinary incontinence. Tumors along the base of the skull (the clivus) present with cranial nerve deficits. Tumors about the pituitary will compromise endocrine function, and may produce a chiasmal syndrome (bitemporal hemianopia). Meningiomas are commonly found along the sphenoid wing and falx. Each pathology has its favorite ecologic niche in the intracranial compartment, so that the experienced clinician can infer the microscopical identity from symptoms and signs.

Tumors of the Hemispheres

The malignant glioma is the most common tumor of the cerebral hemispheres. Men with this tumor outnumber women, and the typical age of onset is 40 to 60 years. The doubling time is short, the duration of symptoms prior to diagnosis of this aggressive tumor is usually less than 3 months. These tumors are sometimes diffusely infiltrating or (apparently) multicentric in the white matter of the hemispheres. Because of their infiltrating nature and origin in the deep white matter, they can grow quite large before disturbing cortical function. The CT scan may reveal a large enhancing lesion with extensive mass displacement at a time when the patient looks relatively well (Fig. 9-12). The other characteristic feature of the malignant glioma is the brain edema it evokes. Dramatic clinical improvement often follows the treatment of surrounding vasogenic brain edema with corticosteroids.

With malignant gliomas (grade III or IV) the median survival of untreated patients is less than 6 months. The introduction of radiation and experimental chemotherapy has more than doubled median survival, though the quality of survival is often poor in the late months. The ability to kill this tumor with radiation is limited by the radiation tolerance of the surrounding normal brain. A dose of radiation that delivers two logs of tumor reduction (6,000–7,000 rad) causes damage to the brain in a substantial percentage of individuals.

Meningiomas are firm, encapsulated tumors which arise in the meninges and invade the brain parenchyma from outside. While they are histologically benign, they may be very difficult to resect and may be ultimately lethal. Cushing's monograph on the meningiomas discusses favored sites for these tumors: adjacent to the dura in the sylvian fossa, along the sagittal sinus, along the olfactory groove and sphenoid wing. They grow very slowly, often invading the dura or venous sinuses, or provoking an osteoblastic reaction in the cranial vault. Plain skull films may provide a clue to diagnosis by showing a suggestive sclerosis of the skull in an otherwise asymptomatic individual. Arising from outside the brain proper, these tumors derive their blood supply from the external carotid via the middle meningeal artery or the meningohypophyseal vessels. Intrinsic glial tumors, on the other hand, are perfused off the local cerebral circulation. This is the basis for the distinction between these tumors by angiography. Meningiomas progress slowly, and those that grow superficially along the convexity in symptomatic individuals can generally be excised for cure.

Posterior Fossa Tumors

Posterior fossa tumors are particularly dangerous because they are likely to block the fourth ventricular outflow channels and cause obstructive hydrocephalus. The medulloblastoma is a tumor of primitive

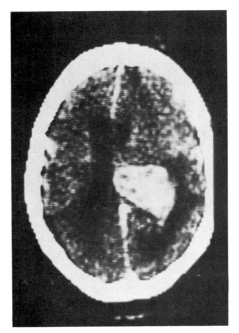

A

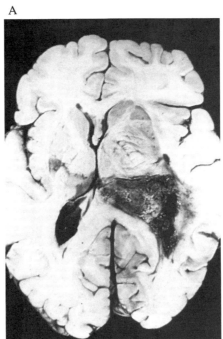

B

cerebellar nerve cells, most common in childhood. Like other anaplastic tumors, it is approached with radiation and chemotherapy with varying success. Meningiomas and acoustic neuromas occur in the posterior fossa in adults. Both are histologically benign, and may be resected if the anatomy is favorable. The acoustic neuroma, a Schwann cell tumor at the cerebellopontine angle, has a clinical syndrome so stereotyped that its presentation should be learned. The patient presents with gradually progressive hearing loss in one ear. Vertigo occurs in a minority of cases, and is often slight or absent. Headache is often a feature. Dysmetria develops (ipsilateral to the hearing loss) as does a disturbance of balance and gait, as the cerebellum is affected. The neighboring cranial nerves are involved: the fifth first, and then the seventh. Loss of the corneal reflex may be an important clue. Long tract signs and hydrocephalus are features of longstanding or advanced disease. Modern diagnostic tests (magnetic resonance imagining, CT, auditory evoked potentials) make confirmation of diagnosis routine at an early stage. The differential diagnosis of a mass in this region includes cholesteatoma or abscess at the cerebellopontine angle.

Pituitary Tumor

Pituitary adenoma can come to attention because of progressive visual loss, endocrine symptoms, or the incidental discovery of destructive enlargement of the sella turcica on skull x-ray or CT. Compression of the optic chiasm typically produces a bitemporal hemianopia, which may be complete or partial. Thirty to forty percent of pituitary tumors produce no hormone, though glycoprotein hormone subunits have recently been identified in many of these cases. Prolactin adenomas are the largest group of hormone-producing tumors. They can present with amenorrhea-galactorrhea, or with infertility. They can sometimes be suppressed medically with dopamine agonists. (Recall that dopamine is prolactin inhibiting factor, or PIF). Acromegaly and Cushing's disease are caused by secretory pituitary adenomas. As a tumor in this region grows large, the rest of the gland may not function. Pituitary tumors sometimes outgrow their blood supply, leading to acute necrosis or "pituitary apoplexy."

FIGURE 9-12. A. Computed tomography scan with contrast shows an enhancing mass in the white matter of the right hemisphere, extending into the corpus callosum, with surrounding edema and shift of midline structures. B. Postmortem section from the same patient shows corresponding tumor, a glioblastoma, with hemorrhage, necrosis, and displacement of surrounding structures.

TABLE 9-5. Site of Primary Tumor from
572 Patients with Intracranial Metastases

Primary Tumor	Brain Metastases Patients (%)	Leptomeningeal Metastases Patients (%)
Lung	61 (26)	34 (15)
Breast	33 (14)	42 (18)
Melanoma	50 (21)	35 (15)
Leukemia	10 (4)	48 (21)
Lymphoma	4 (2)	34 (15)
Testes	17 (9)	3 (1)
Neuroblastoma	2 (1)	6 (3)
Renal	11 (5)	2 (1)
Other	47 (20)	27 (11)
Total	235 (100)	231 (100)

Source: L. Weiss, H. Gilbert, and J. Posner (eds.), *Brain Metastases*. © 1980 by Year Book
Medical Publishers, Inc., with permission.

METASTATIC CANCER

With the increasing success of treatments for systemic cancer, neurologic complications are becoming quite common. In a referral center, one in four patients dying of systemic cancer will have intracranial
or spinal metastases. Intracranial metastases can involve the skull or
dura or can seed the meninges, but they most often present, singly or
multiply, in the brain itself.

  Most carcinomas are bloodborne; they reach the brain by hematogenous spread. Thus pulmonary lesions are frequently present, and
lung cancer is a common source of cerebral metastases. Metastatic
deposits found in the intracranial compartment are reviewed in Table
9-5. Seventy-five percent of cerebral metastases are multiple. They

FIGURE 9-13. Spinal cord compression from extradural tumor. A. Normal
cross-section anatomy of the thoracic spine illustrates the relationship of
the spinal cord (SC) and dura mater (DM) with the vertebral body (VB).
Note the position of the exiting segmental nerve (SN) with regard to the
vertebral body and the posterior elements. SG = spinal (dorsal root) ganglion; DR = dorsal root. Parts of the vertebra: L = lamina; P = pedicle; SP
= spinous process. PM = paraspinal muscles. Note fat and venous plexus
in the epidural space (ES). B. Metastatic tumor usually begins in the vertebral body (VB) and invades the epidural space anteriorly, compressing the
nerve root and/or spinal cord. (From L. Rodichok and G. Harper, Spinal
epidural metastases. *Curr. Concepts Oncol.* 2 : 11–20, with permission.)

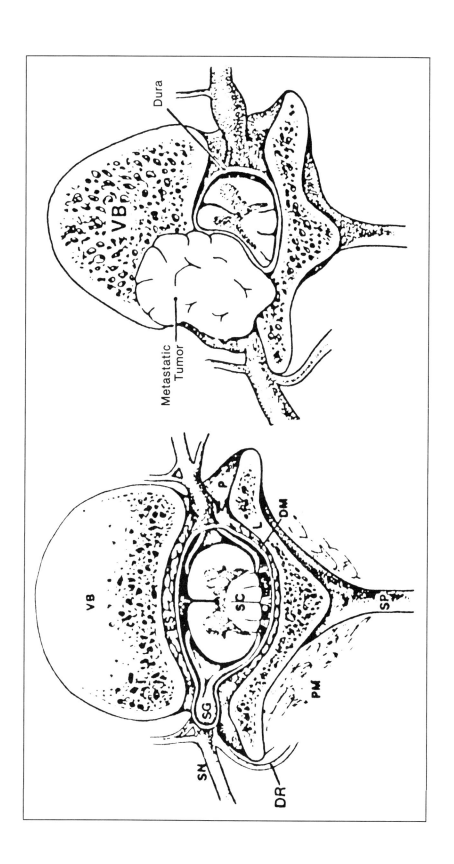

typically invade the rich perivascular space at the base of the cortical ribbon. Some anaplastic tumors with poor cell adhesion characteristics are found in the brain with surprising frequency. Melanoma and germ cell tumors are in this group. Other tumors, such as endometrial cancer, bladder cancer, and prostate and colorectal cancer, uncommonly go to brain. Because metastatic lesions disrupt the integrity of the blood-brain barrier, contrast-enhanced CT scanning is a sensitive diagnostic test. Ninety-five percent of symptomatic lesions will be imaged by this technique, as will some unsuspected metastases.

Some metastatic lesions are sensitive to radiation, and the results are much better than for malignant glioma. A smaller dose of radiation (3,000–4,000 rad) will provide palliation of symptoms for most patients. Most die from their systemic disease, rather than neurologic involvement.

Spinal Cord Compression

Another common complication of cancer is spinal cord compression. Ninety percent of spinal metastases enter the epidural space from a focus in the adjacent spine (Fig. 9-13). Sometimes tumors grow through the neural foramina from the adjacent retroperitoneum. Rarely a focus of tumor can reach the Virchow-Robin space directly from the circulation, and cause an intrinsic metastasis. Space constraints are greater in the spinal canal than in the intracranial compartment, and a mass of 5 to 10 cc will compromise the spinal cord. The syndrome of spinal compression can progress to completion over 24 to 48 hours, making this a true oncologic emergency. Despite use of steroids and radiation treatment, only a small number of patients who present with paraplegia can be restored to ambulatory status.

Leptomeningeal Carcinoma

Any systemic neoplasm can colonize to the meninges, but lung cancer, breast cancer, lymphoma, and leukemia are the most common. The condition usually occurs in the context of prolonged treatment of systemic disease with chemotherapy. As most antineoplastic drugs do not cross the blood-brain barrier, the CNS is a protected place where tumor cells can find safe harbor. Once they break through the endothelial barrier, they establish a focus for meningeal spread (see Fig. 9-3, B). Neoplastic cells may collect in the caudal sac, or in the meninges around the base of the brain. They may congest the arachnoid granulations to promote hydrocephalus. Presenting features include mental status changes and/or scattered segmental deficits from nerve root involvement. Classic signs of meningitis are usually absent. The CSF, as reviewed above, shows a reaction with elevated protein and pleocytosis. Cytologic examination of CSF will commonly reveal tumor cells. Repeated lumbar punctures are sometimes necessary to secure the diagnosis.

BIBLIOGRAPHY

Cushing, H. *Intracranial Tumors.* Springfield, Ill.: Thomas, 1932.

Cushing, H. *The Meningiomas.* Springfield, Ill.: Thomas, 1938.

Fishman, R. Brain edema. *N. Engl. J. Med.* 273 : 706–711, 1975.

Fishman, R. *Cerebrospinal Fluid in Diseases of the Nervous System.* Philadelphia: Saunders, 1980.

Goldstein, G., and Betz, A. The blood-brain barrier. *Sci Am* 255 : 74–83, 1986.

Langefitt, T.W. Summary of the First International Symposium on Intracranial Pressure. *J. Neurosurg.* 38 : 541–544, 1973.

Plum, F., and Posner, J. *Diagnosis of Stupor and Coma.* Philadelphia: Davis 1972.

Posner, J., and Chernik, N. Intracranial metastases from systemic cancer. *Adv. Neurol.* 19 : 579–592, 1978.

Ropper, A., Kennedy, S., and Zervas, N. *Neurological and Neurosurgical Intensive Care.* Baltimore: University Park Press, 1983. Pp 7–21.

CHAPTER 10

Cerebral Metabolism, Brain Ischemia, and Stroke

In this chapter we consider the brain from the perspective of its circulation and metabolic needs. An understanding of the composition and metabolism of nervous tissues is necessary to make sense of the new technologies for brain imaging, such as computed tomography (CT), positron emission tomography (PET), and magnetic resonance imaging (MRI). After a brief review of the cerebral circulation and its regulatory control, the problem of brain ischemia is considered. Stroke is the commonest cause of acquired neurologic deficit in adult life. Migraine is reviewed as a cranial pain syndrome with altered vasomotor activity.

CEREBRAL METABOLISM

The brain is only 2 percent of the body mass, yet it receives 15 percent of the cardiac output and is responsible for 20 percent of the oxygen consumption. The brain expends 49 ml/min of oxygen in the utilization of 77 mg/min of glucose. This metabolic activity is quite high, when compared on a gram-per-gram basis with the heart, liver, or kidney. Brain metabolic activity proceeds at a fixed rate, showing only slight variations with activity and state. Awake or lightly sleeping, daydreaming, or pondering differential equations, the brain steadily consumes substantial quantities of glucose and oxygen. Only extreme conditions such as general anesthesia or a seizure will cause a large change in cerebral metabolism (Table 10-1).

For what purpose does the nervous system expend energy? With the exception of the primary olfactory afferents, nerve cells are postmitotic in adult life. Energy derived from cerebral metabolism is not needed to support growth, and only a small amount is needed for structural maintenance, remodeling, and repair. The brain does not

TABLE 10-1. Cerebral Blood Flow and Metabolic Rate: Variation with Activity

Activity	Cerebral Blood Flow	Cerebral Metabolic Rate
Mentally active	Unchanged	Unchanged
Drowsy or light sleep	Unchanged	Unchanged
Stage IV sleep	Decreased	Decreased
Barbiturate coma	Decreased	Decreased
Anesthesia	Decreased	Decreased
Seizures (during ictus)	Increased	Increased
Anemia	Increased	Unchanged
Hypoventilation, CO_2 rebreathing	Increased	Unchanged

do mechanical work, osmotic work, or extensive synthetic work. Some energy is expended in the synthesis of peptides and neurotransmitters, and in maintenance of the synapses. Axonal transport of proteins made in the cell cytoplasm is moderately costly to nerve cells which maintain lengthy axon processes. The largest share of energy expenditure (about 50%) occurs in relation to synaptic transmission. Another 20 to 30 percent is exhausted in the maintenance of excitable membranes for nerve impulse conduction. A concentration gradient of Na^+ and K^+ ions is maintained by the membrane-bound, adenosine triphosphate (ATP)–dependent pump. This mechanism allows the extrusion of sodium, the sequestration of potassium, and the maintenance of the resting potential.

Glucose is virtually the only substrate for cerebral energy metabolism. It is transported into the brain by a form of facilitated diffusion. Glucose is metabolized to pyruvate in the cytoplasm. Some lactate is generated in the brain, but aerobic metabolism of glucose is required to meet the large energy demands of this tissue. Eighty-five percent of the pyruvate so generated enters the mitochondria for oxidation via the Krebs cycle. Several Krebs cycle metabolites are used as precursors for neurotransmitters: acetylcoenzyme A (acetyl-CoA) for acetylcholine, α-ketoglutarate for glutamate and γ-aminobutyric acid (GABA), oxaloacetate for aspartate. Amino acids cannot be metabolized as fuel by the brain to any appreciable extent. Pyruvate, lactate, and glycerol can be used by nervous tissue in in vitro preparations, but these substances do not penetrate the blood-brain barrier and cannot be extracted for "food." After long periods of starvation, the brain can use keto acids as an energy source. For practical purposes, however, the organ is dependent on the active aerobic metabolism of large amounts of glucose.

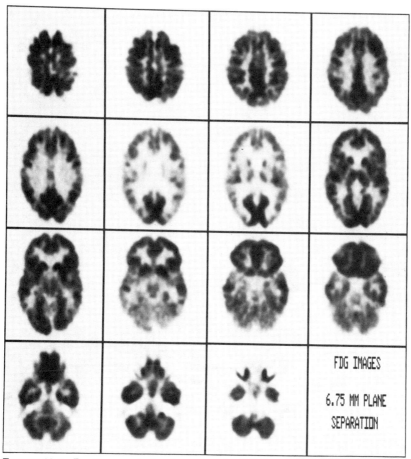

FIGURE 10-1. Positron emission tomography (PET) scan of the normal human brain at rest using ^{18}F deoxyglucose. Greatest metabolic activity is observed in the basal ganglia, thalamus, and neocortex. (Scan courtesy of UCLA Medical Center, Los Angeles, and Siemens Medical Systems, Inc., Des Plaines, Ill.)

Although there is little variation in whole-brain glucose utilization during activity, there are appreciable regional differences in metabolism. New techniques have made it possible to study regional metabolism in laboratory animals. Positron emission tomography has extended these techniques to human subjects. Figure 10-1 shows regional mapping of brain metabolism by PET scan using fluorodeoxyglucose. As might be expected, gray matter is metabolically active relative to white matter. Nuclear groups with the highest metabolic rate at rest include the brainstem and thalamic nuclei of the auditory

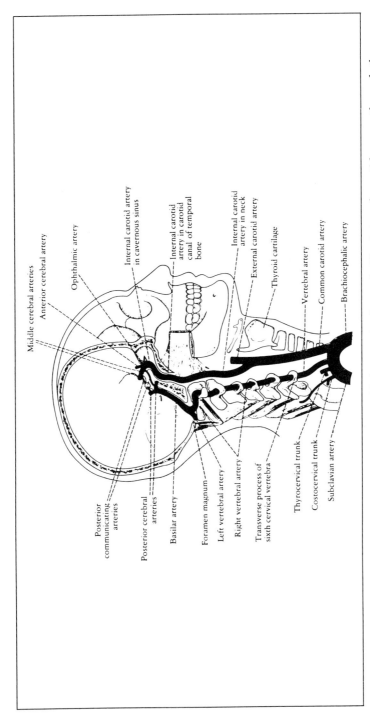

FIGURE 10-2. The carotid circulation. The common carotid bifurcates in the neck. The internal carotid passes through the cavernous sinus, and gives off the ophthalmic artery before it reaches the circle of Willis. The external carotid artery is a source of collaterals about the orbit. (From R. Snell, *Clinical Neuroanatomy for Medical Students* [2nd ed.]. Boston: Little, Brown, 1987, p. 508, with permission.)

and visual system, the basal ganglia, and visual cortex. Regional increases in energy metabolism in the motor cortex can be seen with limb use, and are dramatic after induction of a focal seizure.

Metabolic Encephalopathy (A Brief Reprise)

Brain functions may be disturbed if the nervous system labors under ischemic conditions, or if there is substrate deprivation (hypoglycemia). A number of electrolyte and metabolic abnormalities adversely affect neuronal performance. Metabolic encephalopathy is usually manifest as acute confusion (delirium) or depressed consciousness (see Chap. 6). A variety of disorders can produce this clinical picture: hyponatremia, hypercalcemia, hypercapnia (CO_2 retention), diabetic ketoacidosis, renal failure, and hepatic failure are common examples. Febrile patients often become delirious, while hypothermic patients can be lethargic. Hypothyroidism impairs cerebral function (myxedema madness), as do a number of inherited disorders of amino acid metabolism.

Certain environmental metals, notably lead and mercury, adversely affect brain function. Vitamin and cofactor deficiencies can cause a form of metabolic injury by their impact on substrate utilization. Vitamin B_{12} deficiency is known to affect myelination and impair function in peripheral nerve, spinal tracts, and cerebral white matter. Thiamine deficiency can cause a particular focal necrotizing encephalopathy affecting the hypothalamus, medial thalamus, and oculomotor nuclear groups in the periventricular brainstem. This disorder (Wernicke's hemorrhagic encephalopathy) can be precipitated by the administration of glucose to a patient whose body is depleted of thiamine. Malnourished chronic alcoholics are particularly at risk.

INTRACRANIAL CIRCULATION AND CEREBRAL BLOOD FLOW

Four vessels supply the intracranial compartment: the two carotid arteries; and the two vertebrals, which merge to form the basilar artery. Branches of these main arteries are interconnected by the circle of Willis. The carotid circulation is illustrated in Figure 10-2. The common carotid bifurcates at the level of the thyroid cartilage, giving rise to the internal and external carotids. The internal carotid has no branches in the neck; it enters the cranial vault through the foramen lacerum. After it zigzags through the cavernous sinus, it gives rise to the ophthalmic artery, penetrates the dura, and gives off the anterior choroidal and posterior communicating arteries. When the anterior

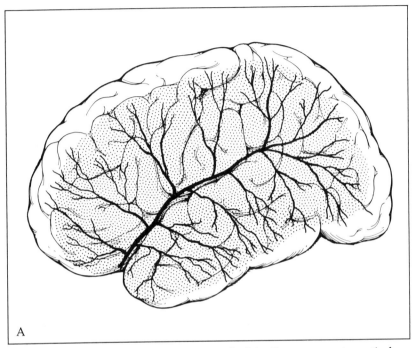

FIGURE 10-3. The middle cerebral artery. A. Stippling represents cortical territory of distribution. Territory includes the sylvian fossa, and adjacent portions of the frontal, parietal, and temporal lobes. B. Penetrating branches supply the basal ganglia and internal capsule. (Modified from R. Snell, *Clinical Neuroanatomy for Medical Students* [2nd ed.]. Boston: Little, Brown, 1987, pp. 510, 511, with permission.)

cerebral artery departs, the trunk that remains is designated the middle cerebral artery. The external carotid is a source of collaterals via its facial and superficial temporal branches. (These anastamose about the orbit with branches of the ophthalmic.) Together, the carotid branches are sometimes referred to as the anterior circulation.

The middle cerebral artery provides blood supply to the lateral convexity of the cerebral hemisphere. Its territory includes the sylvian fossa, the face, arm, and trunk area of the sensorimotor homunculus, and adjacent portions of the frontal, parietal, and temporal lobes (Fig. 10-3). Proximal penetrating branches from the M1 segment near the circle of Willis supply the basal ganglia. The anterior cerebral artery runs a medial course along the corpus callosum (Fig. 10-4). It supplies the medial frontal lobe, the cingulate gyrus, and the anterior

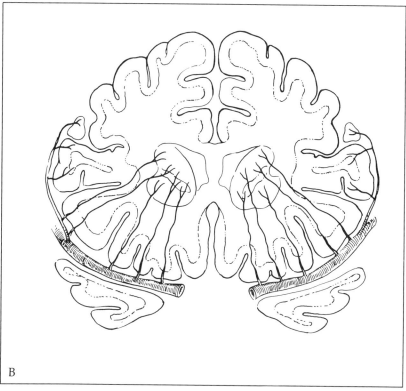

B

FIGURE 10-3 (Continued).

portion of the corpus callosum. Its territory includes the leg area of the
primary motor and somatosensory cortex, and the supplementary
motor area.

The Posterior Circulation

The vertebral artery is the first branch off the subclavian. It tunnels
through the transverse process of cervical vertebrae C5 to C2, and
penetrates the dura at the level of the foramen magnum. Intracranial
branches supply the upper spinal cord, medulla, and the cerebellum
(via the posterior inferior cerebellar artery). At the pons, the two
vertebral arteries merge to form the basilar, which runs the length of
the pons along the clivus. Long circumferential branches (the anterior
inferior cerebellar and superior cerebellar arteries) supply the cerebellum, and penetrating branches supply the basal and medial pons

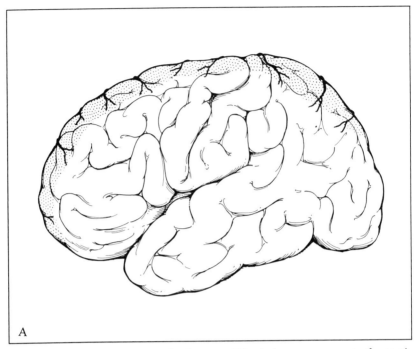

A

FIGURE 10-4. The anterior cerebral artery. Stippled area represents the territory of distribution in lateral view (A) and medial view (B). Territory includes the medial surface, and the anterior four-fifths of the parasagittal convexity and the corpus callosum.

(Fig. 10-5). The basilar artery bifurcates at the midbrain into the two posterior cerebral arteries. Proximal branches of the posterior cerebral supply the midbrain and thalamus. Cortical divisions provide blood supply to the occipital lobe, inferior temporal lobe (including the hippocampus and amygdala), and the posterior fifth of the corpus callosum (Fig. 10-6).

Cerebral Blood Flow

The brain receives 15 percent of the cardiac output, roughly 800 ml/ min. Under ideal circumstances, blood flow should be regulated or precisely tailored to meet metabolic demand. Matching the circulation to metabolism achieves the greatest economy. The precision necessary to match energy consumption and avoid deficits is beyond the capabilities of the systemic circulation, so a special regulatory mechanism has evolved to defend cerebral blood flow.

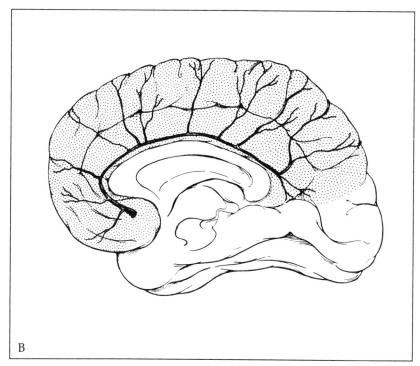

B

FIGURE 10-4 (Continued).

In the systemic circulation, arterial pressure is regulated by a series of cardiovascular reflexes. The baroreceptor reflex is perhaps the most important, sensing arterial pressure at the carotid sinus and aortic arch. There is some reflex neural control of the cerebral circulation as well, but it is much less important. The sympathetics are a weak influence on intracranial vasomotor tone. For the most part, the cerebral circulation is under regional metabolic control (autoregulation). Local control is primarily an effect of acid products of metabolism (lactate, CO_2) on cerebral blood vessels. Conditions that result in local acidosis in nervous tissue cause a compensatory vasodilation, increasing regional cerebral blood flow. Hypoxic conditions also produce local vasodilation and enhanced regional blood flow. Carbon dioxide diffuses across the blood-brain barrier to establish equilibrium. Since HCO_3^- is the largest buffer, the CO_2 tension in nervous tissues determines the local pH. The relationship between cerebral blood flow and CO_2 partial pressure (P_{CO_2}) is illustrated in Figure 10-7. Hyperventilation can reduce P_{CO_2} to around 20 mm Hg in healthy

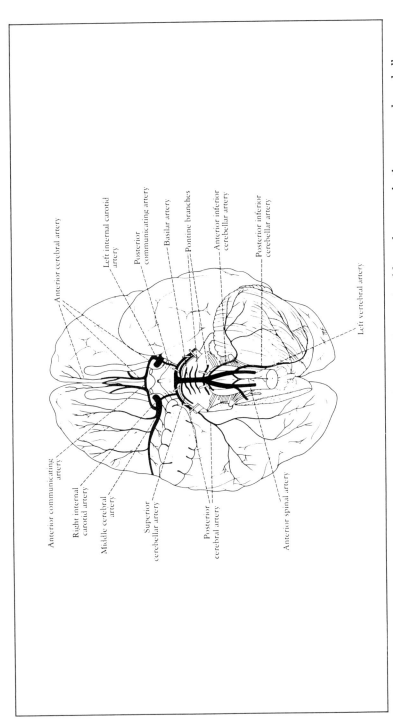

Figure 10-5. Two vertebral arteries merge to form the basilar artery. Its proximal branches supply the pons and cerebellum. (From R. Snell, *Clinical Neuroanatomy for Medical Students* [2nd ed.]. Boston: Little, Brown, 1987, p. 509, with permission.)

Anterior cerebral artery

Left internal carotid artery

Posterior communicating artery

Basilar artery

Pontine branches

Anterior inferior cerebellar artery

Posterior inferior cerebellar artery

Left vertebral artery

Anterior communicating artery

Right internal carotid artery

Middle cerebral artery

Superior cerebellar artery

Posterior cerebral artery

Anterior spinal artery

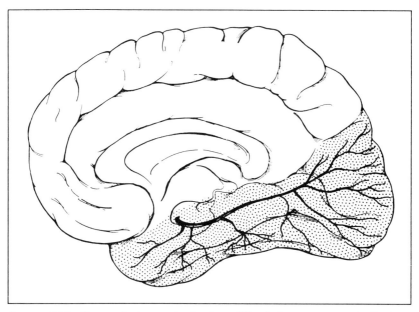

FIGURE 10-6. The posterior cerebral artery. Stippled area represents the territory of distribution. Territory includes the hippocampus, inferior temporal lobe, the occipital lobes. Proximal penetrating branches supply the midbrain and lateral thalamus.

normal subjects, causing a mild alkalosis. The induced vasoconstriction with reduction in cerebral blood volume is enough to effect a modest decrease in intracranial pressure.

Autoregulation controls cerebral vascular resistance and blood flow across the broad range of normal blood pressure variation. Cerebral blood flow is roughly constant between 60 and 150 mm Hg. Outside this normal range, myogenic control of cerebral blood vessels is inoperative and the vessels take a passive role. The relationship between cerebral blood flow and arterial pressure then becomes more linear (Fig. 10-8). The physiologic plateau is known to be shifted to the right (the higher range) in chronically hypertensive patients.

In *hypertensive encephalopathy*, extreme high blood pressure breaks through the upper end of the range of autoregulation. A disturbance in blood flow is associated with extravascular transudation of fluid and brain edema. Headache occurs, with advanced retinopathy, seizures, and signs of raised intracranial pressure.

Autoregulation is also ineffective in patients with cerebral injury due to trauma, hemorrhage, or ischemic stroke. These patients will revert to the passive, near-linear relation between cerebral blood flow and arterial pressure. Attempts to manipulate cerebral blood flow and

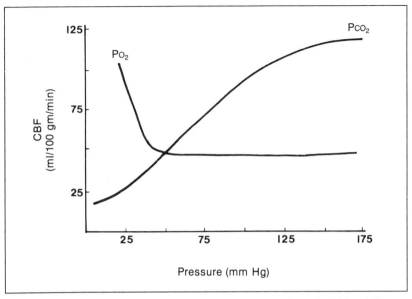

FIGURE 10-7. Cerebral autoregulation: the response of cerebral blood flow (CBF) to changes in the arterial concentration of oxygen and CO_2. Under hypoxic conditions, blood vessels dilate and CBF is increased. Increased PCO_2 from cerebral ischemia also induces an increase in CBF. Hyperventilation (low PCO_2) causes vasoconstriction, reducing cerebral blood flow and blood volume.

blood volume in these patients for therapeutic purposes are often frustrated by the lack of local metabolic control. Such patients are also more vulnerable to hypotension.

BRAIN ISCHEMIA

The brain does not well tolerate interruption of its blood supply. Total cessation of cerebral blood flow results in a loss of consciousness in 5 to 20 seconds. Irreversible tissue injury begins to occur 4 to 8 minutes after total interruption of blood flow. Ischemia seems to be more injurious than oxygen deprivation per se, though they usually occur in combination. If cerebral perfusion is maintained, the brain will tolerate moderately severe degrees of hypoxia (PO_2 20–40 mm Hg) for as long as 30 to 40 minutes. Ischemia may be global, as observed during cardiac arrest, drowning, or exsanguination. Brain ischemia may also be regional, as observed with athero-occlusive cerebral infarction (stroke).

Cerebral blood flow is normally 800 ml/min, roughly 53 ml/100 gm tissue per minute. There is a generous safety margin in normal perfu-

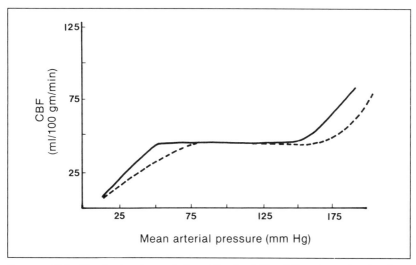

FIGURE 10-8. Cerebral autoregulation: Cerebral blood flow is maintained at a steady level over a broad range of systemic blood pressure, due to myogenic control of cerebral blood vessels. In chronically hypertensive individuals, the range of autoregulation may be shifted (*dotted line*), such that moderate degrees of systemic hypotension reduce cerebral perfusion.

sion. When the regional blood flow drops below 25 to 30 ml/100 gm/min, symptoms are often observed. There is inadequate oxygenated blood to meet metabolic demand. Below 18 ml/100 gm/min, tissue remains viable, but a profound functional disturbance (*electrical failure*) is observed. There is a cessation of brain electrical activity: attenuation of the electroencephalogram (EEG) and absence of cerebral evoked potentials. Below 10 ml/100 gm/min, there is loss of ATP and critical compromise of ion transport. Irreversible injury ultimately ensues. This level of hypoperfusion is called *ionic failure*, as ATP-dependent transport of Na^+ and K^+ is compromised. Potassium leaks out into the extracellular space, and intracellular Ca^{2+} accumulates. Excessive entry of calcium into the neuron is destructive. There is some amount of intracellular acidosis as well, due to anaerobic metabolism of glucose to lactate. After 3 to 4 hours of hypoperfusion at this level (sooner if the perfusion is less), changes become irreversible and cell death results. The problem of severe (sustained total) circulatory failure may be compounded by changes in the microcirculation. An increase in vascular resistance sometimes impedes reperfusion.

The cellular pathologic findings of ischemic neuronal injury are fairly consistent. In stained sections, the cell body of the damaged neuron becomes shrunken and darkly pigmented. As neuronal cells are lost, glial cells proliferate. Under conditions of global ischemia, areas distal in the circulation are hypoperfused. This failure is evident

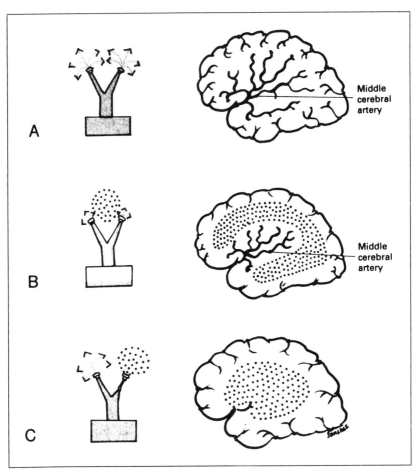

FIGURE 10-9. Circulatory failure and watershed infarction. *A* illustrates the normal state of the circulation, in which the middle cerebral artery provides blood flow to much of the lateral convexity. In *B*, hypotension results in border zone ischemia. Blood goes to the central area of distribution, and stippled areas have poor flow. In *C*, the main stem of the middle cerebral artery is obstructed, and infarction occurs in the artery's core territory. (From L.R. Caplan and R.W. Stein, *Stroke: A Clinical Approach*. Stoneham, MA: Butterworths Publishers, 1986, with permission.)

in the posterior hemisphere at the border zone between the middle and posterior cerebral arteries, and also at the border between the middle and anterior cerebral artery territory (Fig. 10-9). This pattern of distal field or "watershed" infarction is observed in patients with severe hypotension. There are also entire populations of neurons selectively vulnerable to ischemic injury. The pyramidal cells of the hippocampus, especially in CA1 (Sommer's sector), are consistently damaged in cases of severe ischemic injury.

There is some evidence that glutamate plays a role in ongoing neuronal injury during whole-brain ischemia. The mechanism of glutamate toxicity was reviewed in Chapter 5. In ischemic tissues, glial mechanisms for high-affinity glutamate uptake may not function adequately. Neurons contain a large "metabolic pool" of glutamate within them, and liberation of glutamate by dying neurons perpetuates the cycle of cell injury and death. Rothman and Olney, and Choi have demonstrated that retinal neurons or nerve cells in tissue culture can be protected from some of the effects of ischemia by pretreatment with γ-glutamylglycine or AP5, drugs that block the N-methyl-*d*-aspartate (NMDA)–type glutamate receptor. NMDA receptors are found in high concentration in the sector of the hippocampus that is vulnerable to ischemia (CA1). In animal studies, occlusion of the anterior circulation for 2 hours results in an ischemic necrosis of brain with cell loss approaching 60 to 70 percent in some regions. Pretreatment (or early postexposure treatment) with an NMDA receptor blocker substantially reduces the severity of cell death.

Focal Ischemia

Focal ischemia, as observed during stroke, is a more complex problem. While there is no direct circulation through the vascular occlusion, there is often some collateral flow. This results in the delivery of glucose during anaerobic conditions, favoring the formation of lactic acid and severe local tissue acidosis. Often perfusion drops below 10 ml/100 gm/min in a core territory, resulting in ischemic necrosis. Some of the surrounding brain tissue may be too ischemic to function, while remaining critically viable. This tissue, receiving between 10 and 20 ml/100 gm/min, is known as the "ischemic penumbra." Stroke therapy is often directed at the rescue of marginal ischemic tissue, by improving acidosis and oxygen delivery. Calcium channel and NMDA receptor blocking drugs are being explored as well to prevent further loss of neurons. The local disorder of autoregulation may be severe. Ischemic arterioles fail to respond physiologically to the acidosis, while adjacent normal vessels dilate. This disorder of autoregulation results in a shunting of blood flow away from the ischemic zone, and "luxury perfusion" of adjacent tissue. There is a marked tendency for ischemic, acidotic brain tissue to develop edema, which may be observed as an area of low density on the CT scan (Fig. 10-10).

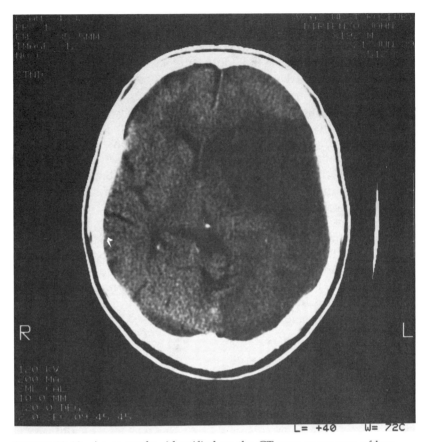

FIGURE 10-10. Acute stroke, identified on the CT scan as an area of low density due to infarction and brain edema. Stroke is in the territory of the middle cerebral artery. There is considerable mass effect, with displacement of midline structures. (CT scan courtesy of Dr. Hani Haykal, VA Medical Center, West Roxbury, Mass.)

STROKE MECHANISMS

The term *stroke* describes the acute onset of a focal neurologic deficit due to vascular disease. Stroke is the third leading cause of death in developed countries. Its annual incidence in North America is 150 to 200 per 100,000 population. In the past decade, there has been some decline in the incidence of stroke, probably related to better control over the principal risk factor: *hypertension*.

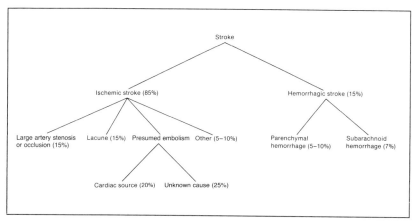

FIGURE 10-11. Principal categories of stroke. Figures in parentheses list approximate relative incidence of stroke subtypes (averaged from various clinical series).

There are two principal mechanisms for stroke: ischemia and hemorrhage. Ischemic strokes account for roughly 85 percent of the total, and a number of major subtypes have been described (Fig. 10-11). In about 20 to 30 percent of ischemic stroke cases, the exact mechanism cannot be defined. Hemorrhagic strokes are almost evenly divided between parenchymal (intracerebral) hemorrhage and subarachnoid hemorrhage. Hemorrhage causes a deficit by dissection and mass effect, though ischemia and edema are often present to some degree as well. A small number of primary intraventricular hemorrhages are also described.

Large Artery Athero-Occlusive (Thrombotic) Stroke

Atherosclerosis has favorite sites of occurrence along the major cranial vessels. The carotid bifurcation is a typical location for large, complex plaques of the type which progress to occlude flow. The internal carotid usually collects the larger deposit. Sometimes narrowing is observed in the carotid siphon. Both are areas of complex alterations in laminar flow. The vertebral is usually affected at its origin, or intracranially at its merge, near the origin of the posterior inferior cerebellar artery. The midbasilar sometimes develops an atherosclerotic narrowing. Factors influencing the evolution of atherosclerosis in cerebral vessels include hypertension, diabetes, and hyperlipidemia.

The capacity of the collateral circulation is an important determinant of the outcome when occlusion develops. Naturally occurring collateral channels are adequate to prevent stroke in many patients as the carotid narrows. There are frequent patients who come to post-mortem examination with a carotid occlusion completely asymptomatic during life. For other patients, the outcome is a large and catastrophic stroke. Symptoms are typically observed when there is narrowing of the luminal area by greater than 90 percent.

As an atheroma blocks the last bit of residual blood flow, a number of events occur to cause regional brain ischemia downstream. Clot propagation may cause flow to fall below the 10 to 15 ml/100 gm/min needed to sustain nervous tissue. Bits of thrombus may break off and lodge in smaller vessels (artery-to-artery embolization). For some patients, intraplaque hemorrhage may be the event which initiates critical flow reduction.

Thrombotic stroke has several characteristics that aid in diagnosis. Onset is commonly stepwise and stuttering, rather than smoothly progressive. The deficit may progress to maximal over 24 to 48 hours in the anterior circulation, or for up to 72 hours in some cases of basilar occlusion. Sixty percent of patients describe prior warning episodes. These are known as *transient ischemic attacks (TIAs)*. Most typically 10 to 30 minutes in duration, TIAs can last up to 24 hours. (By convention of definition, anything longer is a small stroke.) Those in the carotid circulation produce symptoms of focal cerebral or retinal ischemia, while posterior circulation TIAs usually produce a brainstem syndrome. These minor episodes are commonly, but not invariably, a warning of impending stroke.

Embolic Stroke

Embolic stroke is caused by a fibrin thrombus which migrates through the bloodstream and becomes impacted in the cerebral circulation. Studies suggest that this is a very common stroke mechanism; embolism is perhaps underrecognized as a cause of stroke. The heart is the usual source for thrombotic material, but the great vessels sometimes produce embolic fragments, and venous thrombus can rarely enter the arterial circulation through a patent foramen ovale (paradoxical embolus). In 40 to 50 percent of cases, the source for an apparently embolic stroke cannot be determined (even after postmortem examination!).

Once in the cerebral circulation, 80 percent of emboli go to the middle cerebral artery. The remaining 20 percent enter the posterior circulation, many ending up at the top of the basilar or in the posterior cerebral artery. The anatomy and idiosyncracies of the flow pattern produce this distribution of events. Embolic occlusion causes ischemia, the severity of which depends on the collateral circulation. Embolism is a dynamic process; the clot fragments lyse and migrate. By 72 hours it is often difficult to find pieces of embolus on cerebral angiography. Sometimes a proximal branch occlusion will produce an area of ischemia and infarction, then migrate distally to lodge in another branch. This opens perfusion to an ischemic bed. If the injury is substantial to vascular endothelium, reperfusion can convert a bland infarct into one with petechial hemorrhage or focal bleeding (hemorrhagic infarction).

The clinical profile often helps establish a diagnosis in embolic stroke. The deficit is sudden, and usually maximal at the time of onset. The patient may be active at the time of the ictus; some embolic strokes occur during urination or while straining at stool. Occasionally a two-step onset is described. A proximal embolus with mild diffuse ischemia migrates distally, producing a smaller area of dense infarction. In the case of an embolus of cardiac source, the risk can be related to the nature of the underlying heart disease. Rheumatic valvular disease with atrial fibrillation carries a high risk, and is a very common source. Mural thrombus after myocardial infarction is another common source. Some prosthetic valves carry a high risk of systemic (including cerebral) embolization. A few uncommon diseases present with cerebral emboli and are important to recognize, such as atrial myxoma and bacterial endocarditis.

Lacunae

Small infarcts or lacunae ("lakes") are described in relation to occlusive disease of smaller end arteries. These penetrating arteries are 100 to 400 μm in diameter. As described above, they are found off the circle of Willis, the middle cerebral stem, and the vertebrobasilar circulation. Atherosclerotic thrombosis may occur in small vessels at their origin in very hypertensive patients. More typically, occlusion is due to lipohyalinosis—a thickening of the distal vessel wall related to chronic hypertension.

The infarcts vary in size from 2 to 3 mm to over 1 cm. The effect depends on the location. They may be clinically silent. Four or five common lacunar syndromes were described by Fisher, in relation to sites in the internal capsule, thalamus, and basis pontis. Multiple lacunae (état lacunaire) or ischemic change in central white matter (Binswanger's disease) has been described in patients with chronic and severe hypertension.

Other Causes of Ischemic Stroke

This category (miscellaneous) includes a variety of diseases which affect cranial blood vessels or disturb the coagulation process. Arteritis can present with stroke; the optic nerve head is commonly infarcted in temporal arteritis. Dissection of the carotid is described after trauma, and a few cases of vertebral artery dissection have been observed after chiropractic manipulation. Fibromuscular dysplasia can cause carotid stenosis. Changes in blood viscocity (polycythemia) or a hypercoagulable state can also lead to stroke. Disorders of proteins S, C, and a circulating lupus anticoagulant have been associated with stroke. Rarely, thrombosis of the venous system is seen, especially in cancer patients. The result is ischemia and hemorrhagic infarction.

Intracerebral Hemorrhage

Like lacunar infarction, intracerebral hemorrhage is usually a consequence of chronic hypertension. The hemorrhage develops in small penetrating arteries, the same vessels affected by lipohyalinosis. Pathologic examination suggests that hemorrhage may originate with rupture of small Charcot-Bouchard aneurysms which are sometimes present in these vessels. Intracerebral hemorrhages are typically found in relation to this end-arterial circulation. The caudate, putamen, and internal capsule are the most common sites (40–50%), followed by the thalamus (20%), pons, cerebellum, and hemisphere white matter.

The clinical syndrome of intracerebral hemorrhage varies with the location. A steadily progressive onset is typical. There is often vomiting, and there may be headache or signs of raised intracranial pressure with larger hemorrhage. The CT scan is an excellent instrument for diagnosis, as heme iron in blood has high density to x-ray (high signal attenuation). The CT scan in Figure 10-12 shows a small hemorrhage in the medial thalamus, which presented with mild confusion and amnesia. While the larger hemorrhages usually progress to stupor, coma, and death, small hemorrhages cause restricted damage and are compatible with a good outcome.

Lobar intracerebral hemorrhages are increasingly common in the elderly. In these patients, there is often no background history of hypertension. The stroke literature suggests that these hemorrhages may be due to amyloid change in cerebral blood vessels, a pathology associated with Alzheimer's disease and with normal aging. In some

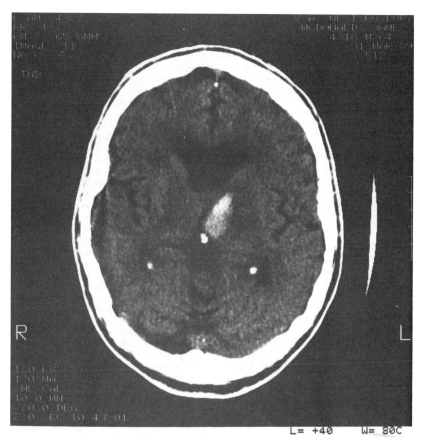

FIGURE 10-12. Intracerebral hemorrhage in the medial thalamus on the dominant side. Blood is dense, and shows up as a region of high signal attenuation (white) on CT scan. (Courtesy of Dr. Hani Haykal, VA Medical Center, West Roxbury, Mass.)

individuals with *cerebral amyloid angiopathy,* multiple hemorrhages have been seen.

Subarachnoid Hemorrhage

Bleeding into the subarachnoid space usually occurs from the rupture of a saccular aneurysm or arteriovenous malformation. Aneurysms are most commonly found in arteries of the circle of Willis. The typical locations for saccular aneurysm are shown in Figure 10-13. They are observed post mortem in 5 percent of the population and many of

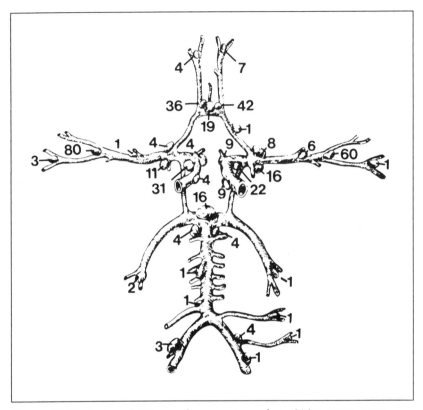

FIGURE 10-13. Series of 429 saccular aneurysms from 316 autopsy cases, with location illustrated in relation to the circle of Willis. Ninety percent occur off the anterior circulation. (From F. McCormick, Vascular Diseases. In R.N. Rosenberg et al., *The Clinical Neurosciences*, Churchill Livingstone, New York, 1983, vol. 3, p. 38, by permission.)

them are unruptured. The saccular aneurysm is often regarded as a congenital defect, but the aneurysm emerges in adult life. A defect is present in the vessel's elastic lamina, most often at bifurcations. During the early decades of life the media thins, the vessel wall expands, and muscle is replaced by fibrous tissue. As a result, the tensile strength of the vessel wall is diminished (Fig. 10-14). Most patients are in their forties or fifties when the aneurysm ruptures.

The risk of hemorrhage is related to aneurysm size, and is probably greatest for those between 7 and 15 mm in diameter. Hypertension is an independent risk factor (think of the inflation of a balloon as a model). The actual bleeding is very brief, but blood spurts out at arterial pressure and the event is fairly destructive. Patients describe the abrupt onset of a severe headache, typically the worst headache of

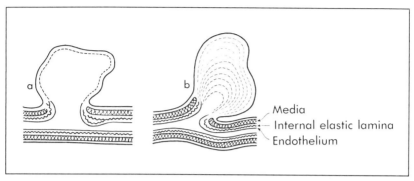

FIGURE 10-14. Diagrammatic representation of the structure of an intra-
cranial aneurysm. Saccular aneurysm in *b* has thrombus within. (From
R. Escourolle and J. Poirier, *Manual of Basic Neuropathology.* Philadelphia:
Saunders, 1973, p. 110, with permission.)

their life. The onset often occurs during vigorous activity. Because the
high pressure interferes with cerebral perfusion, there is sometimes a
transient loss of consciousness. Some patients are fortunate to come
to medical attention with warning symptoms, related to the mass
effect of the aneurysm, or a minor leak (sentinel headache).

Twenty-five to thirty percent of aneurysmal hemorrhages are immediately fatal (or the patient never regains consciousness). There is
a 50 percent 1-year mortality associated with a ruptured aneurysm.
Most of the mortality after the first day is due to rebleeding or "delayed deterioration." Ischemia from vascular spasm is the usual cause
of delayed deterioration. Components of clotted blood promote
vasospasm in animal models. Spasm is often found adjacent to collec-
tions of blood in human patients (as defined by comparing CT with
cerebral angiography).

Approach to Stroke Diagnosis

The process of stroke diagnosis is an exercise in applied anatomy
and clinical reasoning. A diagnosis is usually fashioned in two parts.
First, the information about symptoms and clinical signs is analyzed
to infer the *anatomic localization.* The localization can often be specified
in terms of the vascular anatomy. Then the history is reviewed: the
risk factors, and the nature of the stroke onset. This information,
together with the anatomic localization, is used to make an *etiologic
diagnosis.* Brain imaging tests and other laboratory data are often used
as supporting evidence. Computed tomography, as described above,

is highly useful in the separation of hemorrhagic from ischemic stroke.

As an example, consider the case of a 58-year-old man with atrial fibrillation and rheumatic valvular disease, who develops the acute onset of headache and fluent aphasia. He has had no prior transient symptoms. Examination shows slight asymmetry of the face, no limb weakness, and normal sensation. Visual fields reveal a partial defect in the right upper quadrant. Detailed mental status examination shows that the patient is awake and alert. He produces a stream of paraphasic speech, with no apparent comprehension. Step 1 of the process of diagnosis is to localize the lesion. Fluent aphasia points to the posterior left hemisphere; Wernicke's aphasia occurs with a lesion in the superior temporal gyrus. The involvment of the inferior loop of the optic radiations is consistent with this localization. The stroke is largely cortical, in the territory of the inferior division (trunk) of the middle cerebral artery. Step 2 is to synthesize all the clinical information into an etiologic diagnosis. The abrupt and maximal onset is suggestive of embolus. The branches of the middle cerebral artery are common sites of embolic stroke. Isolated Wernicke's aphasia is due to embolic stroke in 80 to 90 percent of cases. A CT scan would be useful to exclude a small hemorrhage. (This kind of inference can be modeled on a computer as a rule-based expert system.)

MIGRAINE

Migraine is a common disorder affecting cerebral blood vessels. In contrast to stroke, migraine generally has a rather benign course. Estimates suggest that 5 to 10 percent of the population is prone to vascular headaches of the migraine type. Headaches usually begin in adolescence or early adult life. They are hemicranial (involve one side of the head) and throbbing, and are often associated with nausea. Classic migraine is heralded by an aura: neurologic symptoms which precede the headache. Frequently reported migraine auras include scintillating lights obscuring vision, zigzag lines, hemianopia, or migrating paresthesias.

Harold Wolff studied the pain sensitivity of the cranial contents in the 1940s. He stimulated various structures in the intracranial compartment during open neurosurgical procedures. The brain itself is surprisingly insensitive to pain. High sensitivity was encountered in the dura, venous sinuses, and proximal arterial tree. Arterial dilation produces dramatic headache, sometimes experienced by patients taking nitroglycerin or other potent vasodilator drugs. These observations led to the idea that migraine is primarily a disorder of vasoregulation.

The older, generally accepted theory views migraine as a biphasic phenomenon. In the early (prodromal) phase, there is vasospasm. This may be severe enough to produce symptoms, due to regional ischemia. The next event is vasodilation, which results in the headache. Data suggest that circulating vasoactive substances may play a role in the initiation of the attack. (Serotonin levels fall at the onset. Histamine and prostaglandin injections can evoke an attack. Platelet release reactions are increased during the prodromal phase.) Ergotamine, a potent vasoconstrictor, is useful in the treatment of migraine headache for many patients. Cerebral blood flow studies confirm oligemia during classic migraine attacks, with flow levels as low as 15 ml/100 gm/min. However, vasodilation and hyperemia are also observed. The typical pattern is multiphasic and rather complex.

Recent research into the migraine phenomenon has focused on the neural innervation of cerebral blood vessels. Afferent pain fibers in the wall of the anterior circulation vessels have been traced to the gasserian ganglion. Moskowitz has described a trigeminal-vascular system of innervation. The pseudounipolar cells in the fifth ganglion respond to intraluminal administration of bradykinin or mechanical dilation of arteries. The distal nerve endings contain large quantities of peptides, especially substance P, and the machinery necessary to release them into the blood vessel wall. Activity in these pain neurons can release chemical messengers (peptides) distally. Substance P can *cause* vasodilation and extravasation of plasma into the extravascular space.

An alternative hypothesis proposed by Moskowitz views migraine as an abnormal activation of this trigeminal-vascular system. Activity results in pain referred to the cutaneous representation of the trigeminal nerve, and paroxysmal vascular dilation. The trigger for this phenomenon may be hormonal, biochemical, or neural. One interesting possibility is a depolarization phenomenon unique to neocortex, the *spreading depression of Leao*. This regional cortical event, resulting in release of potassium and local acidosis, spreads radially across the cortex at 2 to 6 mm/min. This spread does not respect connectivity relationships or vascular boundaries, and parallels the evolution of the migraine aura. A profound physiologic change of this type in the forebrain could activate the trigeminal-vascular system. The blood vessel changes, which are such a prominent part of the clinical picture, may be a secondary event.

BIBLIOGRAPHY

Adams, R. D., and Victor, M. *Principles of Neurology* (2d. ed.). New York: McGraw-Hill, 1981. Pp. 529–593.

Caplan, L. R., and Stein, R. W. *Stroke: A Clinical Approach.* Stoneham, Mass.: Butterworths, 1986.

Meldrum, B. S. Excitatory amino acids and anoxic/ischemic brain injury. *Trends Neurosci.* 8 : 47–48, 1985.

Meyer, F., et. al. Focal cerebral ischemia: Pathophysiologic mechanisms and rationale for future avenues of treatment. *Mayo Clin. Proc.* 62 : 35–55, 1987.

Moskowitz, M. The neurobiology of vascular head pain. *Ann. Neurol.* 16 : 157–168, 1984.

Sokoloff, L. Circulation and Energy Metabolism of the Brain. In G. Siegel et al., *Basic Neurochemistry* (3rd ed.). Boston: Little Brown, Pp. 471–495.

CHAPTER 11

Neuroimmunology and Neurovirology

Stephen L. Hauser

The fields of neuroimmunology and neurovirology are often grouped together as a single discipline. This grouping reflects in many ways the current gaps in knowledge of this area, particularly as they relate to the pathogenesis of chronic inflammatory disorders of the nervous system. On the other hand, this grouping also serves to highlight the interdependence of these two areas in determining the biologic consequences of exposure to a virus, and the consequences of immune system activation on the host. On a more practical level, it is worth remembering that a number of important diseases of the nervous system, including multiple sclerosis and acute inflammatory polyneuropathy (Guillain-Barré syndrome), appear to be due to an interplay between a viral infection and a host immune response.

THE MOLECULAR BASIS OF DIVERSITY WITHIN THE IMMUNE SYSTEM

While a detailed discussion of the immune system is beyond the scope of this review (the reader is referred to the excellent monograph by Benacerraf and Unanue), a number of basic concepts are important to this area. The two central requirements for a functional immune system are, first, that the system be able to provide effective defense against threats to the organism both from without (such as infectious agents) and within (such as tumor cells) and, second, that this elaborate system of defense not self-activate. In brief, the system must distinguish self from nonself and respond appropriately.

The immune system is comprised of different populations of cells which subserve distinct functions. Thymus-derived or T cells (so

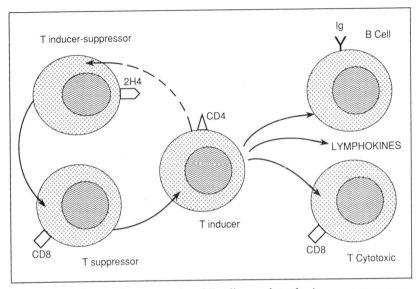

FIGURE 11-1. Interacting networks of T cells regulate the immune response. T inducer cells (CD4 marker) are necessary for B cells to produce immunoglobulin. If sufficient T supressor cells (CD8 marker) are added to B cells and T inducer cells, the production of antibody by B cells is shut off. T inducer cells also produce lymphokines, soluble substances that amplify the immune response and induce T cytotoxic cells. A subgroup of T inducer cells possess the 2H4 marker; these cells are believed to be inducers of suppressor cells.

named because they mature to immunocompetent T cells within the environment of the thymus) are effector cells for specific cell-mediated immune responses including cytotoxic and delayed-type hypersensitivity reactions. T cells also appear to serve important regulatory functions, as demonstrated by their ability to modulate (i.e., induce or suppress) specific immune responses both in vitro and in vivo (Fig. 11-1). B cells, named after the bursa of Fabricius (the organ of B cell maturation in the chicken), are the effector cells for antibody-mediated (humoral) immune responses. The third major cellular element of the immune system is the antigen-presenting cell, or APC, which initiates specific immune responses by "presenting" an antigen, i.e., a molecule capable of stimulating an immune response, to the immune system. APCs are present in the blood as monocytes and reside in most organ systems as tissue macrophages or as other more specialized cells, such as dendritic cells in the skin and microglial cells in the central nervous system (CNS).

Three families of molecules determine, to a great extent, the specificity of antigen recognition by the immune system. They are the immunoglobulin molecule or B cell receptor, the T cell receptor, and the major histocompatibility complex (MHC). These molecules share a degree of homology which suggests that they are derived from the same ancestral gene, and they are frequently classified as members of the "immunoglobulin superfamily" of genes. The immunoglobulin and T cell receptor molecules determine, to a great extent, the specificity of antigen recognition by B cells and T cells, respectively. As noted above, the MHC is required for antigen presentation to T cells and, in ways which remain poorly understood, the MHC also influences whether and to what degree T cells will respond to a particular antigen. In addition, MHC recognition by T cells is essential for cell-to-cell communication (by which T cells direct and modulate immune responses) and for the specific killing of cells by effector or T cytotoxic cells. Elucidation of the genes which encode these three series of molecules and of the mechanisms responsible for diversity of immune responses has been perhaps the most important advance in modern immunology.

The Antigen Receptor on B and T Lymphocytes

The B and T cell receptor genes have evolved a remarkable mechanism whereby enormous genetic information can be contained within a relatively small segment of DNA. In this regard, one of the great questions of immunology, prior to the solution provided by molecular biology, was how diversity, and antibody diversity in particular, was generated. There simply wasn't enough genetic material on the 46 human chromosomes to fit a million different antibody molecule genes. It is estimated, for example, that a total of only 50,000 to 100,000 genes are present in humans. Older theories hypothesized that antigen "instructed" the formation of an antibody molecule which enfolded it (the template theory) or that new specificities were constantly being formed by somatic mutation of DNA, i.e., by mutations which were not contained in germ line DNA. Such theories were inconsistent with known features of the immune response, such as immunologic memory, or with basic principles of protein synthesis (i.e., protein synthesis is directed by nucleic acid and not by antigen). The molecular solution to the problem of antibody diversity was to come, for the B cell receptor, from the laboratory of Tonegawa, and for the T cell receptor, from those of Mark Davis and Tak Mak.

In brief, these molecules are encoded not by an army of individual genes, each containing the entire genetic code for the receptor, but by a series of *gene segment* families which are clustered together on the chromosome. During the process of B cell and T cell differentiation, these gene segments then *rearrange* so that one member of each gene segment family is selected for translation into RNA.

For example, the immunoglobulin (Ig) molecule is composed of two identical light (L) chains and two identical heavy (H) chains. These chains are encoded in three gene families which occur on different chromosomes: λ light chain genes, κ light chain genes, and heavy chain genes. Each L chain gene family is composed of multiple gene segments encoding constant (C), joining (J), and variable (V) regions; H chain genes have an additional group of gene segments called diversity (D) segments. During B cell maturation, rearrangement of the L chain gene complex results in the apposition of a single V gene with a C-J-D complex with deletion of intervening genetic material; similarly, H chain gene complex rearrangement also results in C-J-D-V apposition.

It is not difficult to appreciate how the process of rearrangement contributes to diversity of the immunologic repertoire. For example, the H chain contains 5 different C, 4 J, 12 D, and 200 V gene segments; there are thus 48,000 different H chain possibilities. Similar calculations suggest that there are over 1,200 L chain possibilities. Different combinations between H and L chains would thus result in 6×10^6 different possible Ig molecules.

The T cell receptor (TCR) protein is a heterodimer, or a structure comprised of two different chains (termed α and β) noncovalently associated on the cell surface. As is also the case for the H chain of the Ig molecule, the chain of the TCR is encoded by four gene segments, C, J, D, and V, which rearrange during T cell maturation. Analogous to the Ig light chain, the α chain of the TCR is derived from C-J-V gene segments. In addition to the diversity generated from rearrangements within the TCR, imprecise joining of gene segments as they line up on the rearranged chromosome, as well as somatic mutations within variable gene segments, also contributes to TCR diversity.

In the mouse, alterations in the repertoire of gene segments coding for the β chain of the TCR may be associated with abnormalities of immune function. Thus some mouse strains which are prone to auto-immune disease contain fewer gene segments in either the V or C region. One might speculate that the absence of some rearrangement possibilities in these strains will decrease the repertoire of T cells capable of responding to an antigenic challenge, perhaps increasing the likelihood that a "suboptimal" response, mediated in part by clones cross-reactive with self-determinants, will occur. A central area of investigation in the next few years will focus on an analysis of the TCR repertoire in human immune disorders.

The Major Histocompatibility Complex

The third family of molecules which influences the repertoire of immune system responses are the products of the MHC. The MHC is a gene complex located on chromosome 6 in humans. In ways not completely understood, MHC gene products physically associate with antigen on the surface of an APC and on target cells, and linked recognition of *both* MHC *plus* antigen *by* T cells is a prerequisite for T cell sensitization and for the generation of effector T cytotoxic cell responses (Fig. 11-2). Thus, presentation of antigen by an APC requires MHC expression on the surface of an APC, and MHC expression must be present for a cell expressing a given antigen to be killed by specifically sensitized cytotoxic T cells.

The MHC region in humans (called the *HLA complex*) encodes four loci, termed *HLA-A, -B, -C,* and *-D,* which subserve the above functions, as well as numerous other gene products including several complement genes and genes unrelated to the immune system. The HLA-A, -B, and -C regions correspond loosely to the murine class 1 genes, and the HLA-D region to the class 2 genes originally described in the mouse. Different subsets of T cells interact with different classes of MHC genes. By specifying how antigens are presented to T cells, these genes appear to influence whether or not T cells will respond to particular antigens and how such a response will be regulated. MHC genes may also influence the ultimate T cell repertoire during the course of T cell maturation in the thymus.

Considerable polymorphism or heterogeneity exists among HLA gene products in different individuals, and the presence of specific differences, termed *allelic variants,* is associated in some instances with susceptibility to autoimmune disease. The B27 allele, for example, is strongly associated with ankylosing spondylitis. The largest category of HLA-associated diseases is linked to alleles of the D locus and includes, among others, juvenile-onset diabetes mellitus and lupus erythematosus. Two neurologic diseases associated with alleles of the D locus are multiple sclerosis, which is associated with DR2, and myasthenia gravis, which is associated with DR3. The human D region is now known to contain at least six different genes, and the ability to identify different alleles at each D locus subregion may make it possible to identify more precisely those people at risk for a particular disease. This has recently been accomplished for juvenile diabetes mellitus, where the amino acid specified at residue 57 of the β chain

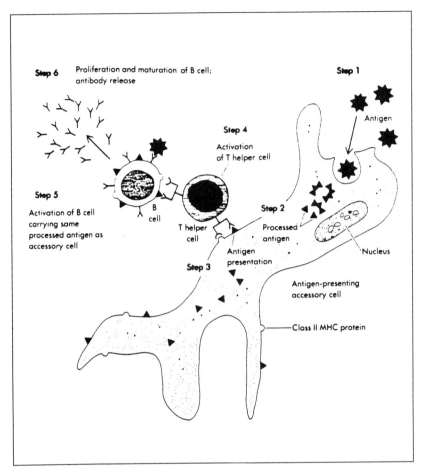

FIGURE 11-2. Amplification of the immune response: antibody production. Antigen is taken up by antigen-presenting cells (APCs) and processed. Fragments of the antigen appear on the surface of the accessory cell. The T helper cell whose antigen-specific T cell receptor can recognize this antigen binds to the APC and becomes activated. The activated T cell then interacts with a B cell whose antibody can recognize the same antigen that stimulated the T helper cell. The B cell also has processed antigen on its surface. The interaction of T and B cells, along with antigen stimulation, triggers the B cell to divide and differentiate to an antibody-producing plasma cell. MHC = major histocompatibility complex. (From L.E. Hood, I.L. Weissman, W.B. Wood, and J.H. Wilson. *Immunology* [2nd ed.]. Copyright © 1984, Benjamin/Cummings Publishing Company, Menlo Park, Calif.)

of a D region locus, termed *DQ*, appears to determine susceptibility to this disease.

The Concept of Idiotypy

An idiotype is the site on the lymphocyte receptor that combines with antigen, and a clone of lymphocytes share a common idiotype. For the B cell receptor, the idiotypic site consists of both H chain and L chain determinants. A single antibody molecule may contain several different idiotypes. The network hypothesis, first postulated by Neils Jerne, states that these idiotypes are themselves immunogenic and, during the course of an immune response, clones of cells are expanded that make anti-idiotypic or antiantigen receptor antibodies. Because the idiotype binds both to the anti-idiotype and to the original antigen, the anti-idiotype may be structurally similar to the original antigen; such anti-idiotypes are said to represent "internal images" of the antigen. In an analogous way, a third-order cell, or an anti–anti-idiotype, may be generated, which may bear a receptor similar to that of the original idiotype (Fig. 11-3).

Jerne postulated that this network of receptor-antireceptor interactions ultimately results in a modulating or regulatory influence on the immune response. While the in vivo significance of immune networks in the naturally occurring immune response remains unknown, it has become clear that manipulation of networks represents a powerful method of modulating the activity of the immune system in an idiotypic-specific manner.

Immune Privilege and the CNS

In 1948, Peter Medawar demonstrated that skin grafts could survive rejection when transplanted to the brain, in contrast to the fate of such transplants in other tissues. Based upon these and similar experiments, the brain has been considered an immunologically privileged site. This relative immunodeficiency of the CNS was thought to reside in the blood-brain barrier which contains vascular tight junctions that under normal circumstances prevent immune cells and most proteins from entering the brain. The absence of a clearly defined lymphatic system within the CNS has also been thought to limit the capacity of the immune system to respond in this organ.

Recent evidence clearly demonstrates that the CNS is not a privileged site for many immune responses. Immune privilege for some (but not all) *primary* immune responses may occur when antigen is

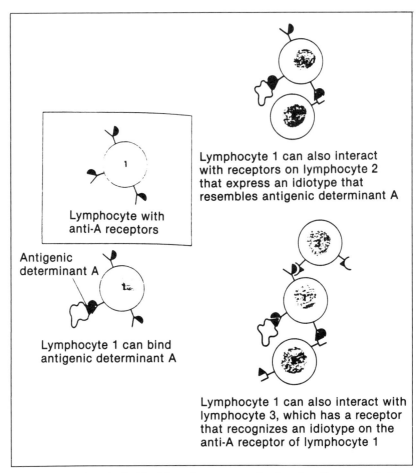

Lymphocyte with
anti-A receptors

Antigenic
determinant A

Lymphocyte 1 can bind
antigenic determinant A

Lymphocyte 1 can also interact
with receptors on lymphocyte 2
that express an idiotype that
resembles antigenic determinant A

Lymphocyte 1 can also interact with
lymphocyte 3, which has a receptor
that recognizes an idiotype on the
anti-A receptor of lymphocyte 1

FIGURE 11-3. Any individual lymphocyte may be functionally connected to other lymphocytes through idiotype–anti-idiotype reactions. There is increasing evidence that such interactions play an important part in regulating at least some immune responses. (From B. Alberts, *Molecular Biology of the Cell.* New York: Garland, 1983, p. 988, with permission.)

presented within the brain of a naive (e.g., unsensitized) animal, but *secondary* immune responses occur efficiently in the CNS in a previously sensitized host. Thus, the CNS may be privileged with respect to the afferent, but not the efferent, limb of the immune response.

T cells can be sensitized to nervous system antigens by peripheral immunization, and in genetically susceptible individuals such cells efficiently cross the blood-brain barrier and mediate a local CNS immune response. Experimental allergic encephalomyelitis (EAE) is an example of an autoimmune disease induced in this way. Susceptible animals, immunized subcutaneously with CNS white matter or with isolated myelin proteins, predictably develop a CNS-restricted inflammatory reaction mediated by T cells and characterized clinically by weakness and ataxia. EAE is widely employed as a model for the human disease multiple sclerosis (see below).

Immune Cell Circulation Within the CNS

Under normal circumstances, mononuclear cells derived from the peripheral blood do circulate within the CNS. This has been most clearly shown for cells of the monocyte-macrophage line which cross the blood-brain barrier and appear in the CNS as macrophages and as microglial cells. In experimental animals, peripheral (usually peritoneal) macrophages are made to phagocytize a marker such as iron filings, and these iron-containing cells can then be found in the CNS. More recently, experimental bone marrow transplant techniques have been used to directly demonstrate that the transplant cell can be identified in the host CNS as a microglial cell. In humans, CNS microglial cells can be labeled using macrophage-specific antibodies.

In normal CNS, small numbers of lymphocytes, generally T cells, are also present. Such cells can also be detected in the cerebrospinal fluid (CSF). It is believed, although not directly proved, that such cells recirculate from the periphery.

A major unanswered question concerns the mechanism by which sensitized T cells in peripheral blood recognize target antigens in the CNS and then cross the blood-brain barrier. Because brain endothelial cells express MHC antigens (see below), it has been postulated that antigens might be presented in association with MHC at the endothelial surface. More recent data suggest that *activated* T lymphocytes may recognize and respond to antigen alone (in the absence of MHC molecules) on the surface of CNS endothelial cells, and that such cells may cross the blood-brain barrier and enter the CNS without participation of MHC molecules. Lymphocyte traffic across venules has, in other organs, been shown to depend upon interaction with an endothelial protein termed *ubiquitin,* and it is possible that other specific receptors for lymphocytes exist in CNS endothelia as well.

MHC Expression in the CNS

Most investigators have not found detectable MHC expression in the normal CNS. For class 1 MHC antigens in particular, this lack of MHC expression is in contrast to that found in most other organ systems, where class 1 expression is easily detected. Endothelial cells and some pericytes express variable levels of both class 1 and class 2 proteins. Microglial cells (which, as noted above, are of hematogenous origin) also express class 2 proteins. Resident CNS cells, including astrocytes, oligodendrocytes, and neurons, appear to express little if any MHC protein under normal conditions. Experimentally, astrocytes can be induced to express large amounts of class 2 antigen when stimulated with the products of activated lymphocytes, and under these conditions astrocytes are capable of serving as APCs and as targets for T cell–mediated cytotoxicity.

It is likely that the low level of class 2 expression in normal CNS accounts for the relative insensitivity of the immune system to the generation of a primary immune response within the CNS. Very low levels of MHC expression, some undetectable by current labeling methods, may be present on the surface of some brain cells, and such cells may be able to serve as targets for T cell–mediated responses; experimentally, this has been shown to be the case for oligodendrocytes.

AUTOIMMUNITY AND THE CNS

Autoimmunity, or loss of immunologic tolerance to self-antigens, appears to be responsible for a number of important diseases of the nervous system, including myasthenia gravis, multiple sclerosis, and acute inflammatory polyneuropathy (Guillain-Barré syndrome). As will become evident from the discussion that follows, many gaps exist in our knowledge of the pathophysiology of these conditions, in particular with regard to the antigens involved in triggering the disease and the exact immunologic mechanisms at work (Table 11–1). As noted above, it is thought that self-reactive T cells are deleted in the thymus, and that susceptibility to autoimmunity may be a consequence of abnormal thymus gland function, or, alternatively, that normal regulatory mechanisms, in particular the generation of T suppressor cells, may fail.

Viral infection has also been implicated in the pathogenesis of some autoimmune diseases. One mechanism of virus-induced autoimmunity might be the generation of an immune response against antigenic determinants shared between virus and the nervous system ("molecular mimicry"). Thus, during the course of an immune response to a virus, antibodies or T cells specific for a viral determinant, might also damage CNS tissue. Other mechanisms to explain virus-induced autoimmunity include virus-induced changes of cell surface components on the cell that the virus infects (such as increased expression of histocompatibility antigens), incorporation of normal tissue components when a virus buds from the membrane of a cell, and direct effects of a virus on immunoregulatory or effector cells leading to non-specific activation of the immune system.

Myasthenia Gravis: a B Cell–Mediated Autoimmune Disease

Myasthenia gravis (MG) is a disease characterized by fluctuating muscular weakness and fatigue. The disease is caused by an antibody-mediated attack against the acetylcholine receptor (AChR). This is a membrane glycoprotein located at the postsynaptic or muscle side of the neuromuscular junction; the AChR binds acetylcholine, the neurotransmitter for motor neurons, and activates depolarization of the muscle membrane initiating contraction.

There are extensive data demonstrating that antibody-mediated dysfunction of the AChR is largely responsible for the signs and symptoms of this disease. The bound antibodies destroy the postsynaptic membrane by a complement-dependent mechanism, they modulate or increase the rate of turnover of surface AChR, and they directly block the binding of acetylcholine by receptor. Perhaps the most striking proof that these antibodies cause MG is the observation that some infants born to myasthenic mothers exhibit a transient form of MG ("neonatal MG") due to the presence of passively transferred antibodies. Antibodies from patients can also passively transfer an MG-like disease when injected into mice.

By using antisera that recognize different determinants on the AChR, it is clear that autoantibodies in MG are directed against a region, called the *major immunogenic region,* located on the extracellular portion of the α chain; this region does not include the ACh-binding site or the site which regulates the ion channel opening mechanism. It appears that only some, and not all, anti-AChR antibodies cause MG and that different determinants of the receptor are recognized by the sera from different patients.

As is the case for most other B cell–mediated immune responses, the autoantibody production in MG appears to be under the control of specifically sensitized T helper cells. It is not yet known whether regulation of the T cell response to the AChR is impaired in MG.

Something must initiate the autoimmune response in MG; two possible clues to this problem are provided by the thymus gland abnormalities characterized by lymphocytic hyperplasia or by histologically diverse thymus gland tumors. In many patients, removal of the abnormal thymus tissue results in clinical improvement in the symptoms of MG. The linkage of thymic abnormalities to an autoimmune attack against the AChR may be through antigens shared between

TABLE 11-1. Autoimmune Diseases of the Nervous System

	Site	Antigen	Mechanism	Trigger
Definite				
Myasthenia gravis	Postsynaptic neuromuscular junction	Acetylcholine receptor (also in EAMG)	Antibody + complement	?Thymic abnormalities
Suspected				
Multiple sclerosis	CNS white matter	Unknown (MBP in EAE)	Unknown (CD4 cells in EAE)	?Loss of suppression; ?virus
Acute inflammatory polyneuritis (Guillain-Barré syndrome)	PNS white matter	Unknown (P2 protein in EAN)	Macrophage stripping of PNS myelin	Viral infection
Neuropathy associated with IgM paraproteinemia	PNS white matter	Myelin-associated glycoprotein	Antibody	Unknown
Acute disseminated encephalomyelitis	CNS white matter	?Myelin basic protein	Unknown	Viral infection
Sydenham's chorea	?Caudate/subthalamic neurons	Unknown	Antibody	Streptococcal infection; ?shared antigen with caudate/subthalamic neurons

Myasthenia (Eaton-Lambert syndrome)	Presynaptic neuromuscular junction	Unknown	Antibody	Tumor in some patients; ?antigen
Paraneoplastic cerebellar degeneration	Cerebellar cortex	Unknown	?Antibody	Tumor; ?shared antigen
Systemic lupus erythematosus	?CNS neurons	Unknown	?Antibody	?Loss of suppression; ?virus
Polymyositis	Muscle	Unknown	Unknown	?Loss of suppression; ?virus

Key: EAMG = experimental allergic myasthenia gravis; CNS = central nervous system; MBP = myelin basic protein; EAE = experimental allergic encephalomyelitis; PNS = peripheral nervous system; EAN = experimental allergic neuritis.

these two structures. Thymic lymphocytes appear to express a surface antigen which cross-reacts with the AChR, and cultured thymic epithelial cells can display musclelike antigens including the AChR. It is possible that AChR-specific T helper cells are generated in the thymus and migrate to the periphery where they promote anti-AChR antibody synthesis.

Patients with MG also have an increase in certain MHC alleles, which may in some way predispose them to the development of autoimmunity. In particular, the alleles B8 and DR3 are common in young female MG patients with thymus gland hyperplasia, and in this group there is an increased frequency of other coexisting autoimmune diseases including thyroiditis, red cell aplasia, and lupus erythematosus.

Multiple Sclerosis

Multiple sclerosis (MS) is a chronic demyelinating disease of the CNS. In most Western countries MS is one of the most common causes of acquired neurologic disability in early and middle adult life, affecting approximately 250,000 Americans. The pathologic hallmarks of MS are inflammation, demyelination and gliosis, or scarring (Fig. 11-4). Myelin is destroyed and replaced with glial scar; the axons which course through affected white matter are, in general, unaffected, although their function is disturbed. The resulting symptoms include sensory complaints, visual loss (due to optic nerve demyelination), motor weakness, incoordination, and incontinence.

The initial event in the development of the MS lesion is believed to be the migration of lymphocytes from peripheral blood into CNS white matter where a focus of inflammation is established. These infiltrating cells are predominantly T cells. Because of the obvious inaccessibility of brain-infiltrating cells, most immunologic research in MS has focused on study of material derived from CSF or peripheral blood.

Characteristic CSF abnormalities in MS patients consist of a mild degree of lymphocytic inflammation (pleocytosis) and elevated levels of immunoglobulin. The first finding correlates with underlying disease activity, whereas the second does not. T cells are overrepresented in the CSF of MS patients compared with their percentages in peripheral blood, and it has been claimed that a small percentage of T cells are activated in CSF when an MS patient is having an acute attack of disease. Although elevated immunoglobulin levels, and the presence of "oligoclonal" immunoglobulin (discrete bands of immunoglobulin separated by differences in migration across an electrical field) are present in most MS patients, these findings are also found in other chronic inflammatory CNS conditions and are thus non-

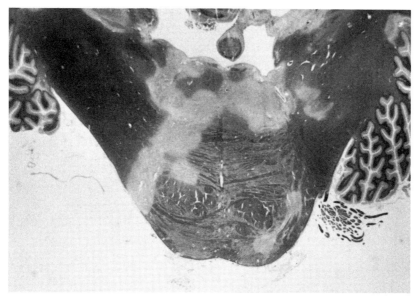

FIGURE 11-4. Section from the brainstem of a patient with multiple sclerosis shows discrete patches of demyelination. Section is stained with luxol fast blue, a reagent that stains myelin. Margins of the demyelinated "plaques" are sharp. Axons are preserved within, but denuded of their myelin sheath. (Courtesy of Dr. James Morris, Brigham and Women's Hospital, Boston.)

specific. The pattern of oligoclonal banding is different for each MS patient, and it is possible that this IgG is produced by random clones of B cells, which are "trapped" in the CNS during the course of disease.

A central question in MS research concerns the antigen against which the autoimmune response is directed. An antigen on myelin or on the myelin-producing cell, the oligodendrocyte, could trigger an immune response resulting in selective demyelination. Much interest has centered on myelin basic protein (MBP), as it has been shown to be the major encephalitogenic determinant for the experimental autoimmune demyelinating disease EAE, mentioned above. Using a variety of different assays, no convincing reactivity to MBP has been identified in MS patients. In fact, in a trial of treatment of MS with injections of MBP, some patients developed a "primary take" to MBP as determined by skin testing. These results suggested that they had not been previously sensitized to MBP. It thus appears that MBP is *not* the target of an autoimmune attack in MS, although it is possible that the appropriate assay to detect anti-MBP reactivity in MS has yet to be developed.

It has recently been found that patients who experience acute CNS demyelination in the setting of measles virus infection (so-called post-infectious encephalomyelitis) do have high antibody titers against MBP in CSF. In several studies, T cell sensitivity to MBP can be measured from CSF or from cells cultured directly from brain tissue of patients with postinfectious encephalomyelitis related to a variety of different viral infections. This disease differs from MS as relapses or a chronic course does not occur.

Epidemiologic evidence does suggest that an environmental exposure, perhaps related to a viral infection, might also influence the development of MS. Clusters and apparent epidemics of MS have been reported, although these reports remain controversial. Early reports of elevated measles antibody titers in the serum of MS patients triggered an interest in the possible role of this virus in MS, and more recently attention has focused on canine distemper virus (a measles-like paramyxovirus), coronaviruses, and human retroviruses (see below). No reproducible demonstration of viral infection in the CNS or MS patients has followed.

A final area of interest concerns the role of genetic predisposition in determining susceptibility to MS. The most compelling evidence in this regard is derived from twin studies. A monozygotic (identical) twin of an MS patient appears to have at least a 50 percent risk of developing MS, compared to a 1 to 2 percent risk for a dizygotic (fraternal) twin or for a nontwin sibling. It is possible that genetic influences are determinants of MS susceptibility either by controlling susceptibility to infection or by regulating the immune response to autoantigen.

Acute Inflammatory Polyneuropathy

Acute inflammatory polyneuropathy (Guillain-Barré syndrome) is an inflammatory demyelinating disease of the *peripheral* nervous system. Pathologically, macrophages penetrate the basement membrane around nerve fibers and strip what appears to be normal myelin from the body of the Schwann cell. In addition to macrophages, perivascular inflammatory cuffs, consisting largely of T cells, are present. Patients with Guillain-Barré syndrome (GBS) typically experience numbness of one or more limbs (often associated with acute neck or back pain) which may then progress to quadriplegia with respiratory insufficiency. Although an ascending paralysis beginning in the lower extremities is the most typical expression of GBS, many variants exist, including descending or localized syndromes, the Miller-Fisher syndrome (ophthalmoplegia, ataxia, and areflexia), pure autonomic insufficiency, and acute neuropathy with severe pain.

Probably the most important etiologic clue to GBS is the finding that a viral infection precedes the onset of the disease in the majority of patients. Many studies have shown an increased incidence of antecedent respiratory infections and gastrointestinal illnesses in patients with GBS, particularly cytomegalovirus, Epstein-Barr virus (EBV), coxsackievirus, echovirus, and the influenza, varicella-zoster, measles, and mumps viruses. Following influenza A/New Jersey virus vaccinations in 1976 and 1977 there appeared to be an increased incidence of GBS, although this has not occurred with other influenza vaccination programs. Some investigators are now questioning whether the association between this "swine flu" vaccine and GBS was real or an artifact. Mycoplasma infection, antecedent surgery, and Hodgkin's disease are also reported to be associated with GBS.

It is striking that a wide variety of infectious agents appear to trigger a stereotyped acute demyelinating disease of the peripheral nervous system. It is unlikely that direct viral infection is responsible for these cases of GBS, as viruses have not been isolated from nerve, and vaccination with inactivated virus may trigger GBS. These agents may act via a common final pathway, perhaps via a shared antigenic structure with the peripheral nervous system or through some as yet undefined common mechanism.

The immunologic mechanism responsible for GBS is not known. A number of experiments have shown that cell-mediated immunity against an as yet undetermined component of peripheral nerve exists in GBS. Recently there has been interest in the participation of humoral factors (e.g, antibody, immune complexes) in GBS, as it has been possible to induce demyelination of peripheral nerve by injecting serum from patients with GBS, and sensitive assays of antibody binding have shown specific antimyelin antibodies in the serum of most patients. It is possible that both cellular and humoral components contribute.

Recent reports suggest that patients with acquired immunodeficiency syndrome (AIDS) and related disorders may have an increased incidence of acute inflammatory polyneuropathy. Because AIDS is associated with hypergammaglobulinemia and with markedly *depressed* cellular immune function, one might speculate whether humoral mechanisms might be responsible for acute inflammatory polyneuropathy in this situation.

IgM Paraproteinemias

The mechanism of neuropathy in some patients with IgM paraproteinemias has been clarified to some degree. It had been previously known that a percentage (approximately 5%) of patients with monoclonal IgM gammopathy developed peripheral neuropathy. In approximately 50 percent of these patients, the monoclonal IgM antibody has been found to react specifically with a glycoprotein of peripheral nerve myelin identified as myelin-associated glycoprotein (MAG). In most patients, the antibodies appear to react with a carbohydrate determinant on MAG. MAG has recently also been found to be present on the surface of a subset of lymphocytes with natural surveillance or natural killer activity, making MAG an example of a shared antigen between the immune system and the CNS. Why this minor protein (constituting less than 1% by weight) of peripheral nerve myelin should be recognized by such a large percentage of paraproteinemias remains totally unknown.

Paraneoplastic Syndromes

In a variety of instances, diseases of muscle (dermatomyositis), nerve (sensory neuropathy, dysautonomia), or CNS (cerebellar degeneration, encephalomyelitis) are associated with tumors elsewhere in the body. Paraneoplastic syndromes are particularly associated with oat cell carcinomas of the lung and with lymphomas.

Recent studies have shown that specific autoantibodies in the serum of patients may play a role in several paraneoplastic diseases. The presence of antibodies against cerebellar Purkinje cells is associated with many cases of cerebellar degeneration associated with malignancy. Patients with the myasthenic (Eaton-Lambert) syndrome, a disease often associated with cancer, have antibodies directed against the presynaptic portion of the neuromuscular junction. Finally, antibodies reactive with retinal neurons have been found in patients with small-cell lung carcinoma who have visual dysfunction.

In these disorders, the mechanisms which generate the autoimmune attack have not been clarified. Although one recent study has shown that a MAG-like molecule is present on small-cell lung tumors, it is clear that shared antigenicity between tumor and normal nervous system tissue is not the only pathophysiologic mechanism to explain the variety of paraneoplastic syndromes known to exist. Examples of other possible etiologies include elaboration of factors from the tumor which then cause nervous system dysfunction, or direct infection by a virus in an immunocompromised host (such as occurs in progressive multifocal leukoencephalopathy).

EXPERIMENTAL MODELS OF AUTOIMMUNE NEUROLOGIC DISEASE

Animal models of autoallergy to nervous system antigens have been of major importance to the study of immune-mediated nervous system diseases. These experimental diseases are induced (or triggered) by injection of the appropriate antigen (or tissue) with an immunostimulator, usually Freund's adjuvant. Thus, experimental allergic MG (EAMG) serves as a model for MG, experimental allergic encephalomyelitis (EAE) for MS, and experimental allergic neuritis (EAN) for acute inflammatory polyneuritis (AIP); these models are summarized in Table 11-2.

EAMG is produced by the inoculation of AChR in adjuvant and is manifested by weakness, with fatigability, reduced miniature end plate potentials, decreased amplitude of the muscle action potential to repetitive stimulation, and clinical response to anticholinesterase medication. Antibody and complement can be visualized by electron microscopy at the postsynaptic portion of the neuromuscular junction. In all of these respects, EAMG appears to be an excellent disease model for human MG. Certain forms of EAMG appear to be mediated by antibody, and animal-to-animal transfer of disease can be accomplished using sera from affected animals. Analysis of AChR-specific autoantibodies in EAMG using monoclonal antibodies has revealed that antibodies are produced against multiple portions of the receptor molecule, and that some antibodies are more important than others in the production of signs of disease.

EAE, first described in 1932, is an inflammatory CNS demyelinating disease. Two recent advances in EAE methodology have resulted in the development of a closer human disease model and have permitted new insights to be gained into the immunologic basis of EAE. In the first, spontaneously relapsing and remitting models of EAE have been described which closely resemble MS both clinically and pathologically. In the second, the recent development of a reliable method of EAE induction in mice has permitted the study of EAE using the tools of murine immunology. Thus, it has now been demonstrated that the T inducer (CD4) cell subset mediates both acute and chronic EAE in the mouse, suggesting that the immunologic mechanism of EAE is that of a delayed-type hypersensitivity response.

Myelin basic protein is known to be an effective antigen for the induction of EAE in most species. As noted in earlier sections, sensitivity to MBP has been difficult to demonstrate in patients with MS, but is present in some patients with acute disseminated encephalomyelitis (ADE) and postinfectious encephalomyelitis; EAE might be a better model for these diseases than for MS. Proteolipid protein (PLP), a major protein component of myelin, is also an antigen for EAE. Recent findings that still other nervous system antigens, alone or in combination with MBP, may induce relapsing EAE have important implications for the study of MS.

TABLE 11-2. Animal Models of Autoimmune Nervous System Diseases

	Experimental Allergic Myasthenia Gravis (EAMG)	Experimental Allergic Encephalitis (EAE)	Experimental Allergic Neuritis (EAN)
Human disease counterpart	Myasthenia gravis	Multiple sclerosis	Acute inflammatory polyneuritis (Guillain-Barré syndrome)
Antigen	Acetylcholine receptor	Myelin basic protein (in some models, proteolipid protein or galactocerebroside)	P2 protein
Mechanism	Antibody + complement	CD4 cells; ?antibody in some models	Sensitized cells; ?antibody in some models
Passive transfer	Serum	CD4 cells	Cells
Analogy to human disease	Excellent	Acute EAE resembles acute disseminated encephalomyelitis more than it does multiple sclerosis (MS); chronic relapsing EAE may be a closer model of MS	Unknown. Pathology of EAN and AIP are similar

The clinical course and pathologic findings of nerve lesions in EAN closely resemble those found in accute inflammatory polyneuritis (Guillain-Barré syndrome [GBS]). The antigen responsible for EAN appears to be a basic protein of peripheral nerve myelin termed P2 protein. Animal-to-animal transfer of EAN requires sensitized T inducer cells, although recently humoral factors have also been implicated in EAN. As previously noted, sensitivity to P2 protein has *not* been found in patients with GBS.

NEUROVIROLOGY

Under natural conditions, the fate of inoculation with a neurotropic virus is, for the host, critically determined by a series of events which occur *prior to* the entry of the virus into the nervous system. These events include the route of entry of the virus into the host, the size of the viral inoculum, the ability of the virus to propagate in a local site prior to distant dissemination, the effect of the host immune system on viral clearance, and the capacity of the virus to penetrate the blood-brain barrier, to name but a few. Initial contact with the host may be through the bite of an insect, such as a tick or mosquito (arthropod-borne or arbovirus), or via the bite of an infected mammal (rabies virus). Some neurotropic viruses enter the host via the respiratory (measles, mumps, varicella-zoster, and herpes simplex type 1) or the gastrointestinal (poliovirus) tracts. Venereal entry is utilized by still other viruses including herpes simplex type 2 and human immunodeficiency (HIV) viruses.

Virus Entry into the Nervous System

The two most frequent pathways by which viruses spread to the nervous system are by hematogenous or neural routes. A hematogenous route has been proposed for viruses such as measles, EBV, and HIV, each of which has the ability to infect circulating lymphocytes. Such viruses may be transported passively across the blood-brain barrier within infected cells (a "Trojan horse" mechanism). Some viruses, such as polio, may infect directly and replicate within brain capillary endothelium, facilitating spread to the nervous tissue. Replication in choroid plexus cells or passage across choroid basement membrane may represent an important route of CNS entry for measles and for eastern encephalitis viruses.

Unlike viruses that enter the nervous system via the bloodstream, rabies virus reaches the CNS by spread along peripheral nerves.

Thus, interruption of peripheral nerves in the vicinity of a rabies virus inoculum prevents the CNS infection characteristic of this virus. Type 1 herpes simplex virus, the virus responsible for the most common nonepidemic encephalomyelitis virus in humans, also enters the CNS via direct neural spread.

Neural Tropism

Once inside the CNS, neurotropic viruses must interact with resident nervous system cells in order to produce pathologic consequences in the host. Viral tropism, against one or several cell types of the CNS, is determined in part by the presence of specific viral proteins capable of binding to surface receptors on target cells. In some instances, the virus may attach via receptors that subserve other functions for the host; thus, host cell receptors for neurotropic viruses may include the AChR for rabies virus, the receptor for the third component of complement for EBV, the CD4 molecule for HIV, the epidermal growth factor receptor for vaccinia virus, and the β-adrenergic receptor for reovirus type 3.

Viral Latency and Persistent Infection

Some viruses have the capacity to produce latent infection in the nervous system. The term *latency* is defined as persistence of the virus genome without production of live virus but with the potential for subsequent virus reactivation. Herpesviruses, in particular herpes simplex type 1 (HSV-1) and varicella-zoster virus, may remain dormant for decades in sensory ganglia. For HSV-1, recurrent activation in the form of cold sores or labial herpes is common, and may be related to section of the nerve proximal to the ganglion, to nonspecific illness, or to stress. This virus is also responsible for a severe, necrotizing encephalitis localized to the orbital-frontal and temporal lobes; the relationship, if any, between latent infection and acute encephalitis has not been clarified.

Examples of diseases due to persistent infection by neurotropic viruses include, in humans, subacute sclerosing panencephalitis (SSPE), progressive rubella panencephalitis, and progressive multifocal leukoencephalopathy (PML). A recently discovered human retrovirus, human T-lymphotropic virus type I (HTLV-I), has been shown to produce a chronic illness reminiscent of MS. Animal models of persistent viral infection, most notably visna virus infection of sheep and Theiler's virus infection in mice, also produce demyelinating lesions similar to those found in MS.

SSPE is a progressive neurologic disease characterized by dementia, motor deficits, and seizures with myoclonic jerking, leading inexorably in almost all cases to death. Measles virus antigen can be identified in brain tissue of affected individuals and live virus can be recovered in some cases. Measles messenger RNA (mRNA) has been identified in neurons, glial cells, and lymphocytes of patients with SSPE. It has been postulated that the synthesis of one measles protein, termed M *protein*, is downregulated, or that the protein itself is defective, and that there is resultant impairment of viral budding from the surface of the infected cell. Patients with SSPE have low or absent titers of antibodies to the M protein, in contrast to high levels of antibodies to other structural proteins of measles. It is also likely that the immune response of the host may influence susceptibility to SSPE.

Infection with Theiler's murine encephalomyelitis virus (TMEV) illustrates the complex interactions between virus and host which may determine the fate of acute infection with a neurotropic virus. TMEV is a murine picornavirus which produces an acute encephalitis with productive viral infection within neurons. In some strains of inbred mice, this acute infection is followed by complete recovery and then by a chronic CNS white matter disease characterized by inflammation, demyelination, and gliosis. These chronic lesions are associated with persistent infection of oligodendrocytes. Different strains of TMEV have been identified which induce only acute disease, only chronic disease, or a combination of the two. Host susceptibility to the chronic demyelinating disease induced by TMEV has been mapped to the MHC of the mouse, and at least one other gene system may also influence the outcome of infection. It is likely that a similar interplay between the genetic background of the virus and that of the host determines the ultimate fate of infection with other neurotropic viruses as well as TMEV.

Progressive multifocal leukoencephalopathy (PML) is characterized by demyelinating lesions throughout the CNS white matter associated with dramatic morphologic changes in glial cells, both astrocytes and oligodendrocytes. Seen almost exclusively in chronically ill or immunosuppressed patients, PML is caused by a papovavirus, either simian virus 40 or a new virus named JC after the patient from whom it was isolated. One of the unusual features of CNS infection with these agents is that no inflammatory response is present in the brains of affected individuals.

Slow Virus Infections of the Nervous System

A group of CNS diseases, typified by Creutzfeldt-Jacob disease and kuru in man and by scrapie in sheep, appear to be caused by a new class of filtrable viruslike agents. Because transmission of infection is sensitive to protease treatment, the term *prion* has been coined to suggest the possibility that an infectious protein might be responsible for these diseases. (Transmission of conventional viruses may also be inhibited by incubation with proteases.) An abnormal sialoglycoprotein, termed PrP 27-30, has been identified in infectious tissue of scrapie-infected animals, but the exact relationship between this protein and the infectious agent remains to be elucidated.

Retroviruses and the CNS

The neurologic consequences of infection with HIV assume increasing importance as the breadth of the AIDS epidemic widens. HIV appears to enter the CNS via infected blood monocytes, and the majority of infected cells in the brains of affected individuals appear to be of monocyte origin. The receptor for HIV on lymphocytes is the CD4 antigen, and it has now been shown that CD4 expression may also be found on human neurons and glial cells. No consistent evidence of HIV infection of these cell types has been found, however, and the pathogenesis of HIV-related neurologic syndromes—including dementia, peripheral neuropathy, and myelopathy—remains unknown.

A second human retrovirus, HTLV-I, is associated, in approximately 1 percent of infected individuals, with a chronic progressive myelopathy which resembles the idiopathic demyelinating disease MS. Little is known at this time about the pathogenesis of this condition, and direct infection of the CNS by this virus has yet to be demonstrated.

The mechanisms whereby retroviruses may persist has been clarified to some extent for the neurotropic sheep virus visna. Visna is a lentivirus which is closely related, in terms of its size and genetic organization, to HIV. Visna virus produces a chronic inflammatory nervous system disease which has also been proposed as a model for MS. It has been shown that new variants of visna virus, which differ generally by single amino acid substitutions in the envelope glycoprotein, are produced continuously during the course of infection. Such new mutants might shield the virus from host immune defenses. In addition, visna may persist in a latent state (as proviral DNA, or DNA complementary to infectious viral RNA) within macrophages, with little or no visna virus protein present at the surface of the carrier cell.

BIBLIOGRAPHY

Alberts, B., et al. *Molecular Biology of the Cell.* New York; Garland 1983. Pp.958–1012.

Asbury, A. K., Arnason, B. G., and Adams, R. D. The inflammatory lesion in idiopathic polyneuritis—its role in pathogenesis. *Medicine (Baltimore)* 48 : 173, 1969.

Benacerraf, B., and Unanue, E. R. *Textbook of Immunology* (2nd ed.). Baltimore: Williams & Wilkins, 1985.

Johnson, R. T. *Viral Infections of the Nervous System.* New York: Raven Press, 1982.

Johnson, R. T., et al. Measles encephalomyelitis—clinical and immunologic studies. *N. Engl. J. Med.,* 310 : 137–141, 1984.

Lindstrom, J. Immunobiology of myasthenia gravis, experimental autoimmune myasthenia gravis, and Lambert-Eaton syndrome. *Annu. Rev. Immunol.* 3 : 109–131, 1985.

McFarlin, D. E., and McFarland, H. F. Multiple sclerosis. *N. Engl. J. Med.,* 307 : 1183–1188,1246–1251, 1982

Tyler, K. L., and McPhee, D. A. Molecular and genetic aspects of the pathogenesis of viral infections of the central nervous system. *CRC Crit. Rev. Neurobiol.* 3 : 221–243, 1987.

Index

Index